D1530480

COMPACT *Research*

Biomedical Ethics

Current Issues

Other books in the Compact Research series include:

Drugs
Heroin
Marijuana
Methamphetamine
Nicotine and Tobacco
Performance-Enhancing Drugs

Current Issues
The Death Penalty
Gun Control
Illegal Immigration
World Energy Crisis

COMPACT *Research*

Biomedical Ethics

by Don Nardo

Current Issues

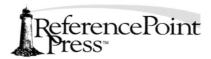
ReferencePoint Press™

San Diego, CA

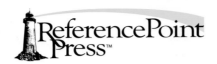

© 2007 ReferencePoint Press, Inc.

For more information, contact:
ReferencePoint Press, Inc.
17150 Via del Campo Road, Suite 204
San Diego, CA 92127
www.ReferencePointPress.com

ALL RIGHTS RESERVED.
No part of this work covered by the copyright hereon may be reproduced or used in any form or by any means—graphic, electronic, or mechanical, including photocopying, recording, taping, Web distribution, or information storage retrieval systems—without the written permission of the publisher.

Picture Credits:
AP/Wide World Photos, 14, 18
Maury Aaseng, 33–36, 48–50, 64–67, 80–82

Series design:
Tamia Dowlatabadi

LIBRARY OF CONGRESS CATALOGING-IN-PUBLICATION DATA

Nardo, Don, 1947–
  Biomedical ethics / by Don Nardo.
    p. cm. — (Compact Research series)
  Includes bibliographical references and index.
  ISBN-13: 978-1-60152-013-5 (hardback)
  ISBN-10: 1-60152-013-1 (hardback)
  1. Medical ethics—Juvenile literature.   I. Nardo, Don
1964–   . II. Title.
R724.N357 2006
174.2—dc22

                                                    2006032649

Contents

Foreword

66 **Where is the knowledge we have lost in information?** 99

—"The Rock," T.S. Eliot

As modern civilization continues to evolve, its ability to create, store, distribute, and access information expands exponentially. The explosion of information from all media continues to increase at a phenomenal rate. By 2020 some experts predict the worldwide information base will double every seventy-three days. While access to diverse sources of information and perspectives is paramount to any democratic society, information alone cannot help people gain knowledge and understanding. Information must be organized and presented clearly and succinctly in order to be understood. The challenge in the digital age becomes not the creation of information, but how best to sort, organize, enhance, and present information.

ReferencePoint Press developed the Compact Research series with this challenge of the information age in mind. More than any other subject area today, researching current events can yield vast, diverse, and unqualified information that can be intimidating and overwhelming for even the most advanced and motivated researcher. The Compact Research series offers a compact, relevant, intelligent, and conveniently organized collection of information covering a variety of current and controversial topics ranging from illegal immigration to marijuana.

The series focuses on three types of information: objective single-author narratives, opinion-based primary source quotations, and facts and statistics. The clearly written objective narratives provide context and reliable background information. Primary source quotes are carefully selected and cited, exposing the reader to differing points of view. And facts and statistics sections aid the reader in evaluating perspectives. Presenting these key types of information creates a richer, more balanced learning experience.

For better understanding and convenience, the series enhances information by organizing it into narrower topics and adding design features that make it easy for a reader to identify desired content. For example, in *Compact Research: Illegal Immigration*, a chapter covering the economic impact of illegal immigration has an objective narrative explaining the various ways the economy is impacted, a balanced section of numerous primary source quotes on the topic, followed by facts and full-color illustrations to encourage evaluation of contrasting perspectives.

The ancient Roman philosopher Lucius Annaeus Seneca wrote, "It is quality rather than quantity that matters." More than just a collection of content, the Compact Research series is simply committed to creating, finding, organizing, and presenting the most relevant and appropriate amount of information on a current topic in a user-friendly style that invites, intrigues, and fosters understanding.

Biomedical Ethics at a Glance

Physician-Assisted Suicide
Legality
Though many Americans feel that physician-assisted suicide is acceptable, Oregon remains the only U.S. state in which the practice is legal.

Religious Objections
One major reason that physician-assisted suicide is so controversial is that Christianity, Judaism, Islam, and most other religions condemn it.

Genetic Testing
Fears
One of the primary worries of opponents of genetic testing is that the procedure might encourage people to manipulate natural processes such as genetic inheritance for bad purposes.

Protecting Privacy
To discourage the use of people's genetic information to discriminate against them, forty-two states have passed laws banning such discrimination by insurance companies.

Human Embryonic Stem Cells
Medical Potential
Some 100 million Americans and about 2 billion people worldwide suffer from diseases that potentially could be cured using stem cell technology.

Federal Funding

In 2006 President George W. Bush vetoed a congressional bill that would have allowed U.S. government funding of embryonic stem cell research.

Cloning
Technological Breakthroughs

Between 1996 and 2006, sheep, cows, pigs, horses, cats, dogs, and monkeys were all cloned, leading many experts to believe that human cloning will occur in the near future.

Legality

Although a few states, including California and Michigan, have banned human cloning, no U.S. federal law against it yet exists.

Overview: Questions of Morality in a Technological Age

> 66 The concept of bioethics gives us opportunities as a global society to examine the whole foundations of technology and adjust it to the direction that society should take. 99

> — Anna Tilley, "Bioethics," *Biomedical Scientist*, June 2001.

Biomedical ethics (or bioethics) is the branch of philosophy and ethics that deals with the life sciences—of which the major ones are medicine, biology, ecology, and genetics—and their potential impact on society and people's lives. Governments, communities, and individuals often question and debate the various issues surrounding these sciences. One frequently debated bioethical issue, for example, is whether doctors should be allowed to assist people who desire to commit suicide. Other hot topics in the realm of biomedical ethics include deciding how long to keep unconscious patients alive on respirators and other machines; ensuring the privacy of patients' medical records; reproductive rights, including the right to have abortions; genetic testing of fetuses and babies; the use of human embryos in stem cell research; and cloning human beings. An enormous amount of disagreement exists over the ethical and moral dimensions of these and other similar issues. For instance, some people object to physician-assisted suicide on religious grounds. Others feel it is a matter of personal liberty and want to see it legalized everywhere. Similarly, some people believe that aborting a fetus is a form of murder, while others think it is not and that women should be free to choose to have an abortion if they wish.

All of these issues involve various aspects of modern scientific and medical technology. Almost every week, some new technological breakthrough occurs in medicine, biology, or one of the other life sciences. And the speed and scope of the onrush of technological advancement is so great that even doctors, never mind ordinary nonmedical laymen, cannot keep up with and fully grasp it all. There is a tendency, therefore, for people to try to control the spread and uses of technology. The common view is that, without some basic rules and safeguards, technology might run amok, as in the famous fictional story of Dr. Frankenstein, who created artificial life with disastrous results. In fact, many people see exerting control over biomedical technology as a matter of social and personal responsibility.

> **Almost every week, some new technological breakthrough occurs in medicine, biology, or one of the other life sciences.**

As one expert puts it:

> Science is one of the most powerful agents of change in our society and we, as the members of that society, need to be able to control it. . . . The concept of bioethics gives us opportunities . . . [to] adjust . . . [technology] to the direction that society should take, rather than the inevitable direction that technology assumes.[1]

Thus, the effort to control biomedical technology almost always brings biomedical ethics and bioethicists into the picture. Bioethicists are individuals trained in the life sciences, philosophy, ethics, and law. They advise doctors, medical researchers, hospitals, politicians, judges, news organizations, community officials, companies, and ordinary citizens on bioethical issues. Religious leaders, politicians, lawyers, and judges also frequently enter the discussion. This is because society, in its efforts to keep the application of technology ethical, often turns to religious teachings or norms for guidance and/or passes laws regulating such application. These norms and laws frequently remain controversial, however. While some people strongly feel that strict societal guidelines are necessary, others view them as too restrictive and counter to individual freedom. For the foreseeable future, therefore, heated disagreement and debate will likely remain a central feature of most, if not all, bioethical issues.

Care of Seriously Ill and Dying Patients

One of the areas of biomedical ethics in which such disagreement and debate is often loud is that involving issues of death, dying, and efforts to save the lives of severely ill patients. For instance, ethical disagreements exist over the use of organs donated for transplant operations. These organs are usually in very short supply. And some people think that allowing the buying and selling of organs on the open market would increase the supply. A majority of people, however, including most bioethicists, think that buying and selling human organs raises serious moral questions. These ethically based opinions have swayed legislators to legally ban the sale of organs. There are also serious disagreements in the medical and legal communities over whether minors should be allowed to become organ donors. The main argument against it is that minors are too young and immature to make such important, life-altering decisions.

> " A majority of people, however, including most bioethicists, think that buying and selling human organs raises serious moral questions. "

Similarly, major arguments periodically erupt over issues relating to euthanasia—ending the life of someone who suffers from a terminal illness or incurable condition. Physician-assisted suicide is one such issue. Some people feel that if they themselves become terminally ill they should have the right to ask a doctor to help them end their suffering. Others are convinced that a doctor who aids in a suicide is committing murder.

Another crucial euthanasia-related issue is whether terminally ill or comatose patients should be kept alive by machines. Ethical questions surrounding the issue include: For how long should a person be connected? At what point is it ethical to disconnect the machines? Who should have the authority to decide such matters? These questions, which both doctors and bioethicists attempt to answer, revolve around the concept of what the medical community calls "futile treatment," or medical measures that have no realistic chance of saving the patient. Medical doctor Chris Rangel believes that in some cases a physician should consider withdrawing treatment if it is in the best interests of the patient. "We are not . . . talking about disposing of those patients we judge to have such poor quality of life as to not be worth living," says Rangel. "Rather we are talking about limiting pain and suffering in patients when the inevitable end is near."[2] The problem is that there is frequently considerable disagreement among doctors, patients' family members, and bioethicists about futility in individual cases. As professors Nancy S. Jecker and Lawrence J. Schneiderman point out:

> People may set different cut-off points regarding how low the odds of success must be for the treatment to be futile. . . . Likewise, there may not be unanimous agreement about what qualities of outcomes are poor enough to qualify as futile.[3]

The Emotional Schiavo Case

Sometimes ethical disagreements about futile treatment burst into the headlines and spark discussions and arguments on a national scale. Indeed, in February and March 2005 the attention of every news agency in the United States, and many around the world, was virtually riveted on the case of a Florida woman named Terri Schiavo. In 1990 she had suffered cardiac arrest and fallen first into a coma and then into a persistent vegetative state. In such a state, a person's brain functions are impaired and he or she is usually kept alive by respirators, feeding tubes, or other medical machines and devices. Seeing no hope that Schiavo would ever recover, in 1998 her husband asked that her feeding tube be removed and that she be allowed to die with dignity. He claimed to base the decision on a prior conversation with his wife; he said she had told him that if she was ever in such a vegetative state she would not want to be kept alive artificially. She had not, however, made this clear in writing.

The patient's parents, on the other hand, felt that there was still a chance their daughter might at least partially recover. So they petitioned the courts to force doctors to keep the feeding tubes in. Eventually the

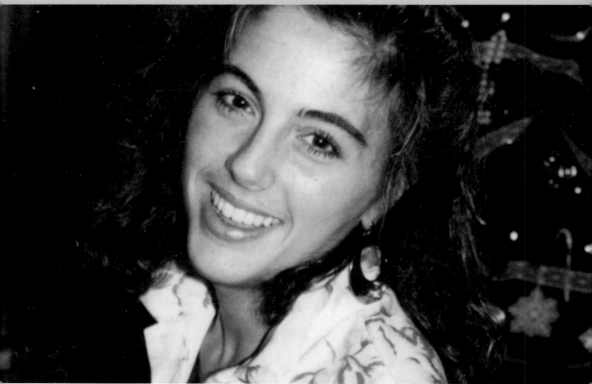

In 2005 Terri Schiavo (pictured before she suffered severe brain damage) was at the center of a heated ethical debate about physician-assisted suicide. On March 13, 2005, her life support system was removed and she died thirteen days later.

state of Florida got involved, and an emotional debate took place in the U.S. Congress; legislators took sides and argued over whether or not allowing Schiavo to die was humane or inhumane, as well as morally right or morally wrong. Some even went so far as to call the proposed removal of her feeding tubes murder. People on each side of the issue cited the views of bioethicists who agreed with them.

Meanwhile, some experts proposed that the case had less to do with ultimate notions of right and wrong and more to do with the patient's own wishes. For example, one of the leading bioethicists in the country, Arthur Caplan of the Center for Bioethics at the University of Pennsylvania, stated:

> It is clear that the time has come to let Terri die. . . . Not because her quality of life is too poor for anyone to think it meaningful to go on. Not even because she costs a lot of money to continue to care for. Simply because her husband

who loves her and has stuck by her for more than 15 years says she would not want to live the way she is living.[4]

Finally, the courts agreed with Schiavo's husband and allowed doctors to remove the feeding tubes on March 13, 2005. She died thirteen days later. Bioethicists across the country continued to disagree over whether she should have been kept alive indefinitely. However, nearly all agreed that one way of avoiding similar tragic and controversial cases in the future would be for each person to make his or her feelings on the matter clear in writing. As noted bioethicist Laurie Zoloth puts it:

> There is one way to make some meaning from this tragic case. . . . Think about what you would wish to do if you were ever in Mrs. Schiavo's condition. Write your wishes down and make a copy for your family. Talk to them about it, talk to your clergy-person about your wishes.[5]

Ethical Questions About Reproductive Issues

The Schiavo case shows how bioethicists can help lead a national discussion of a controversial issue. Such discussions often lead to raised public awareness and sometimes the creation of new approaches to patient care and medical research or new laws regulating these disciplines. But even when ethical issues relating to the life sciences do not make the national news, bioethicists play a part in shaping the way that scientists and doctors deal with these issues.

> **A national discussion of a controversial issue [can] lead to raised public awareness and sometimes the creation of new approaches to patient care.**

Some of the issues surrounding control over human reproduction are clear examples. The most familiar of the reproductive issues is abortion, including arguments over whether it is moral or immoral and whether it should remain legal or be outlawed. These arguments are loudly debated in newspapers, on TV and talk radio, and on the Internet. And bioethicists play prominent roles in these discussions. Covered far less often in the news in recent years are ongoing developments in reproductive technology, such as assisted reproduction and pregnancy reduction; each involves numerous ethical questions that doctors and their patients struggle to answer. As science writer Catherine Baker points out, "Prenatal testing and reproductive technology are giving more people the opportunity to be parents of healthy children. However, along with these opportunities come [ethical] decisions that must be made."[6]

Assisted reproduction is a catchall phrase used to describe medical techniques intended to help people who encounter difficulties in having babies. Among the more familiar of these techniques is the use of fertility drugs, which increase the number of eggs a woman produces. Others include in vitro fertilization (uniting an egg and sperm in the lab and then implanting the fertilized egg into a woman's womb); donation of sperm, eggs, or even embryos by anonymous donors; freezing sperm or embryos for future use; and the use of surrogate mothers.

There is no question that all of these techniques have helped people have children. However, all have also raised ethical questions and dilemmas, many of which have led to court cases. For example, in the case of frozen embryos, arguments have arisen over whether these should be viewed as human beings and who should be awarded custody of them. Some couples who created and froze embryos later got divorced and waged custody battles over the embryos. Similarly, ethical and legal questions have arisen over who has custody when three or even four separate parties are involved. In some cases, eggs and sperm from two anonymous, unrelated donors were procured by a third party; that party then hired a fourth party, a surrogate mother, to carry the baby to term. Bioethicists, lawyers, and judges eventually wrestled over which of the four parties had legal claim to the resulting children; the results varied from case to case, leaving most of those involved feeling unsatisfied.

> **[Reducing pregnancies] inevitably raises the question of whether it is ethical to destroy the lives of some of one's potential offspring in order to ensure the health of others.**

Ethical questions have also arisen in cases of pregnancy reduction, more properly called multi-fetal pregnancy reduction, or MFPR. This relatively new procedure, which began to be performed in the 1980s and 1990s, involves pregnant women who are carrying three or more fetuses and for medical or personal reasons do not want to give birth to them all. Accordingly, a doctor removes one or more of the fetuses, thereby "reducing" the pregnancy. The procedure is most often done in cases of four or more fetuses and between the ninth and twelfth weeks of the pregnancy. Reducing pregnancies is perfectly legal in places where abortion is legal. However, the technique inevitably raises the question of whether it is ethical to destroy the lives of some of one's potential offspring in order to ensure the health of others in the same womb.

Altering the Blueprints of Life

Although pregnancy reduction is not often discussed in public forums such as newspapers and television programs, the opposite is true of several of the ethical issues surrounding the science of genetics. Genetics is a branch of biology that investigates the phenomenon of heredity—the passing along of physical characteristics from one generation to another through DNA and other means. (DNA is a complex chemical composing the genes, the tiny molecular units in the cells of all living things that carry the blueprints for reproduction). In the last two decades geneticists and other researchers have made huge strides in understanding how the genes transmit genetic information from parents to children. The Human Genome Project, begun in 1990 by the U.S. Department of Energy and National Institutes of Health, has so far identified more than twenty-five thousand separate human genes from the total sequence of some 3 billion chemical base pairs in human DNA.

Meanwhile, other researchers began to unlock the mysteries of stem cells (special cells that have the ability to grow into any kind of tissue) and cloning (reproducing a living thing from the genes of a single parent). In 1996 scientists in a Scottish lab cloned a lamb, which they named Dolly; and since that time thousands of sheep, cows, pigs, and other animals have been successfully cloned.

The implications of ongoing genetic research are momentous, both for science and society. Understanding the complex sequence of human genes promises to allow scientists to manipulate genes and thereby to alter the physical traits of new generations of plants, animals, and humans.

Many experts say that stem cell research will lead to the ability to grow new human organs to replace damaged ones. And cloning animals already provides science and industry with improved methods of making certain medicines and breeding more effective research animals.

Just as momentous, however, are the ethical implications of modern genetic research. Some bioethicists, politicians, and religious groups, as well as numerous ordinary citizens, are concerned about the morality of stem cell research, for instance. This is because some people believe that the most promising aspects of the research involve the destruction of human embryos, which the critics view as human life.

Many people are also worried that scientists will succeed in cloning human beings. Among the moral objections voiced against cloning

Reproductive technologies raise many ethical and moral questions. A major concern for some is the potential for genetic enhancement of children, or designer babies. In this picture embryos are carefully transferred from a plastic dish into a special cooler.

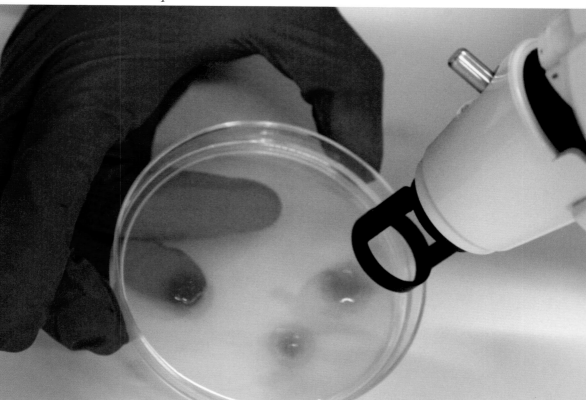

is that doing so is contrary to the natural order of things established by God. As Bill Muehlenberg, national secretary of the Australian Family Association, explains, "Ultimately, cloning is an attempt to play God, to take over his divine prerogatives."[7] However, others disagree, arguing that society does not have the right to prevent an individual from choosing to clone. The Clone Rights United Front, an organization in favor of human cloning, insists, "Each person's DNA is his or her personal property. To have that DNA cloned into another extended life is part and parcel of his or her own right to control his or her own reproduction."[8]

Designer Babies

Another ethical argument to emerge from ongoing genetic research concerns genetic enhancement of children, or the creation of so-called designer children. As one commentator explains:

> At . . . [some] point, it might be possible to manipulate the genes of embryos. Imagine your doctor taking your order: "Okay, that's blue eyes, blonde hair, button nose. And will that be 6 feet 2 inches or 6 feet 4 inches?" The idea of designing our babies is not as far-fetched as it may have seemed just a decade ago.[9]

However, once again ethical arguments arise. Nicholas Agar, a scholar and bioethicist at the University of Wellington, in New Zealand, points out:

> Some of the most challenging moral and ethical questions about a license to design babies concern the societies it might lead to. . . . Will genetic enhancement [create] societies in which unenhanced people are viewed by their genetic superiors in much the same way that we currently view chimpanzees, suitable for drug testing and zoo exhibits but little else?[10]

This is only one of many provocative ethical questions that modern researchers, politicians, and the general public must try to answer in an age increasingly shaped by the onrush of science and technology.

Is Physician-Assisted Suicide Ethical?

"Whichever path society does choose in regards to physician-assisted suicide, moral objections will need to be addressed."

—Andrew D. Boyd, "Physician-Assisted Suicide: For and Against," American Medical Student Association, November 14, 2005.

F ew modern issues have raised more ethical concerns and spawned more debate and legal battles than physician-assisted suicide, often called simply assisted suicide or PAS. Some experts have noted that part of the emotionally charged debate over PAS is about exactly what assisted suicide is. Many people associate it with or call it euthanasia. Euthanasia, or mercy killing, is most often defined as bringing about the death of an ill or suffering person with the intent of ending his or her suffering. The person who commits euthanasia can be a doctor or other health care professional, a family member, a friend, or in theory anyone. Most importantly, that person takes some kind of direct action that ends the patient's life, either with or without the patient's knowledge or permission.

In contrast, in physician-assisted suicide the principal actor is the patient, while a doctor merely provides aid. The American Geriatrics Society defines PAS this way: "When a physician provides either equipment or medication, or informs the patient of the most efficacious [effective] use of already available means, for the purpose of assisting the patient to end his or her own life."[11]

However, in the ongoing societal debate about physician-assisted suicide, the distinctions, between euthanasia and PAS are frequently viewed by some people as mere technicalities. This is because large numbers of people in the United States and many other countries have strong moral objections to both euthanasia and PAS. And they want both to be illegal.

In fact, euthanasia is illegal in the United States, and PAS is illegal in all U.S. states except Oregon. In July 1997 the U.S. Supreme Court upheld laws passed in a number of states making assisted suicide criminal; in October of the same year, Oregon passed its own law allowing doctors to prescribe drugs to people desiring to commit suicide, although the doctors are forbidden from actually administering the drugs. Still, the fact that a majority of people in Oregon favor keeping assisted suicide legal is telling. In fact, polls taken in other parts of the country reveal that large numbers of people in each state have no moral objections to PAS. As a result, physician-assisted suicide remains the subject of periodic and heated debate among health care professionals, legislators, and ordinary citizens.

> **Euthanasia is illegal in the United States, and PAS is illegal in all U.S. states except Oregon.**

Precedents for the PAS Debate

The debate over assisted suicide is far from new. The practice, along with strong opinions both for and against it, existed in the ancient world and is well documented among the ancient Greeks and Romans. Numerous references to doctors aiding their patients in achieving quick, painless deaths are recorded in Roman literature, for instance. Among the most common methods were cutting veins, thereby allowing the patient to slowly bleed to death, and administering drugs or poisons that made the patient lose consciousness.

In contrast, the Greek physician Hippocrates, today considered the father of medicine, objected to assisted suicide. He and his followers banned the practice, as well as introduced the Hippocratic Oath, in which a doctor promised to "do no harm" to patients. Today, doctors across the globe continue to take the oath. And one section of it is often cited by both physicians and medical schools who are opposed to PAS: "I will neither give a deadly drug to anybody, not even if asked for it, nor will I make a suggestion to this effect."[12]

The debate about the morality of assisted suicide continued in the nineteenth and twentieth centuries but did not become the subject of national interest until the 1990s. The controversy was due mainly to the actions of one doctor, a pathologist named Jack Kevorkian. By his own admission, between 1990 and 1998 he assisted nearly a hundred people in taking their own lives. The publicity generated made Kevorkian a household name, and law enforcement authorities tried to prosecute him several times, although they were consistently unable to secure a conviction. In September 1998, however, Kevorkian agreed to appear on the CBS investigative news program *60 Minutes*. During his interview, he allowed the show to air a video of one of his assisted suicides, and the graphic nature of the segment caused a loud public outcry. Authorities soon prosecuted Kevorkian again, this time obtaining a conviction for which he was sentenced to serve ten to twenty-five years in prison.

> " Medical and legal experts say that Kevorkian was not the only doctor or health care professional who performed assisted suicides before and during his years of notoriety. "

Medical and legal experts say that Kevorkian was not the only doctor or health care professional who performed assisted suicides before and during his years of notoriety. Others did so, but in secret for fear of enduring adverse social and legal repercussions. Moreover, this situation has not changed since Kevorkian was convicted. According to reporter Noelle Knox, "Assisted suicide and euthanasia take place in every nation, including in American states where it's illegal."[13]

Arguments in Favor of PAS

It was certainly no coincidence that the U.S. Supreme Court decision against assisted suicide and the passage of Oregon's law for PAS occurred in 1997, at the height of controversy surrounding Kevorkian. His notoriety at the time drew public attention to PAS and stimulated vigorous debate in both public and private circles. And despite the fact that Kevorkian was ultimately convicted and imprisoned, numerous people of all walks of life felt that he was innocent of wrongdoing and offered arguments supporting the morality of assisted suicide.

Among these pro-PAS positions is one that argues that each human being has a right to personal happiness, as well as the right and obligation to try to make his or her family and friends happy. According to this doctrine, which some refer to as "utilitarian morality," under certain circumstances the greater happiness might require the person to take his or her life. Robert B. Mellert, a philosophy professor and noted commentator on bioethical issues, gives the following illustrative scenario:

> I am one who is terminally ill, facing pain and suffering for the rest of my life, and the cost of prolonging my life is wiping out the money I have saved for my children and grandchildren. What if . . . I conclude that . . . to maximize happiness (for my kin) and minimize pain (for myself) warrants my terminating my life? Then the most caring act a doctor can offer me is to assist me in suicide.[14]

Another argument often cited in favor of assisted suicide is that doctors and other health care professionals need to show compassion for terminally ill patients who no longer wish to go on living. Kathryn L. Tucker, director of legal affairs for Compassion & Choices, explains this point of view. She says, "Even with excellent pain and symptom control a fraction of patients will confront a dying process so prolonged and marked by such extreme suffering . . . that they determine that hastening impending death is the least worse alternative."[15] In such cases, says Tucker, the most compassionate course of action is to allow that person to end his or her life.

Personal Autonomy

Perhaps the most often cited argument in favor of physician-assisted suicide is that of personal autonomy, or an individual's right to freedom of choice and decision making. The medical literature is filled with references to cases in which seriously or terminally ill patients requested that their doctors help them end their lives with dignity. One of the more prominent of these cases was that of George A. Kingsley, who filed suit in New York in 1994, saying in part, "It is my desire that my physician prescribe suitable drugs for me to consume for the purpose of hastening my death."[16] However, the courts rejected Kingsley's plea, which was based on the idea that he had the inherent human right to control his own life, including when and how it should end.

Advocates of the concept of autonomy have sometimes likened it to a civil right that must not be abridged by the government. In 1995 a Washington State federal appeals court ruled in favor of this concept, finding that the decision to commit assisted suicide is a constitutionally protected liberty. The Supreme Court later overruled the decision, upholding the old law. PAS advocate Peter Singer echoes the opinion that individuals should have the right to end their own lives if they choose. He says, "Anyone who values individual liberty should agree . . . that the person whose life it is should be the one to decide if that life is worth continuing."[17]

Arguments Against PAS

Although many people view the arguments in favor of assisted suicide as persuasive, many others cite what they see as even more persuasive arguments against PAS. One of the more common anti-PAS positions is that suffering and death are inevitable natural occurrences and that it is not the place of doctors to intervene in nature's affairs. Critic Richard Radtke argues that instead of looking for ways to help people end their lives, doctors should be focused on helping to make the end of life as comfortable and painless as possible. Says Radtke, "There are more options available through medicine today than ever before to make life more comfortable. Let us spend our time, money, and effort working on pain management rather than on ways to hasten death."[18]

Some other arguments frequently directed against assisted suicide are connected to the affairs of medical personnel and their patients. One such argument, for example, is that PAS undermines medical ethics by sending

> "One of the more common anti-PAS positions is that suffering and death are inevitable natural occurrences and that it is not the place of doctors to intervene in nature's affairs."

a wrong and dangerous signal to health care professionals; namely, that it is all right for them to kill someone when they deem it fitting. As medical doctor David C. Stolinsky maintains, "Since ancient times, society assigned the task of saving life to physicians. If killing people was required, that task was given to executioners. Now [with assisted suicide] we have confused these opposite roles."[19] A related argument states that PAS harms the physician-patient relationship. According to this view, if a few physicians decide to cross the line and take their patients' lives, members of the general public may come to distrust most or all doctors. Bioethicists Eric Cohen and Leon R. Kass explain, "If doctors and others are to faithfully benefit the life the patient still has, they cannot sit in ultimate judgment of its worth, and cannot even think that lethal intervention is an acceptable 'therapeutic option.'"[20]

Another medically related ethical argument against assisted suicide, the so-called slippery slope, posits that allowing PAS to become legal and common is likely to lead doctors to commit other forms of killing. Stolinsky insists, "If *all* human life isn't sacred, none is. . . . Who is worthy to live becomes just a matter of opinion."[21] Some people are afraid, for example, that the right to physician-assisted suicide will spread from the terminally ill to the disabled or mentally impaired. Bioethicist Wesley J. Smith argues that this has been the case in the Netherlands, where PAS is legal. According to Smith, "As the Dutch experience clearly demonstrates—[when physician assisted suicide is legalized] it quickly ceases to be rare, nor is killing resorted to only when all else fails."[22] According to Smith, Dutch doctors assist suicides of depressed people in addition to the terminally ill, and practice euthanasia on infants with birth defects.

Religious Arguments Against Assisted Suicide

Still another argument against physician-assisted suicide is that it violates a patient's dignity because it is more dignified for terminally ill people to allow death to take its course according to what some see as God's plan. "God is the author of life," asserts Catholic scholar John B. Feister. "The medical evidence is that, when pain is managed effectively, when depression is treated, people can encounter life's final passage with dignity, in God's hands."[23] Devout Christians are not the only people who object to PAS on religious grounds. In the words of one religiously based organization:

Many faith groups within Christian, Muslim, Jewish and other religions believe that God gives life and therefore only God should take it away. . . . They feel that we are all stewards of our own lives, but that suicide should never be an option.[24]

The fact that nearly all churches and religious organizations in the United States have spoken out against assisted suicide is a revealing indicator of the chances of PAS becoming legal in other states besides Oregon in the near future. Like the medical profession itself, religion is an institution so basic and powerful in American life that few have the inclination or desire to fight it on major principles. Therefore, regardless of how convincing the ethical arguments for legalizing PAS may be to some people, as long as the churches, synagogues, and mosques are against it, legalization will surely be an uphill battle at best.

Is Physician-Assisted Suicide Ethical?

> **To declare that society must give you permission to kill yourself—is to contradict the right to life. . . . Each individual has the right to decide the hour of his death.**

—Thomas A. Bowden, "Assisted Suicide: A Moral Right," Ayn Rand Insititute, January 31, 2006. www.aynrand.org.

Bowden is an attorney and writer for the Ayn Rand Institute, an organization dedicated to promoting the principles of individual rights.

> **Since a patient cannot end his own life without the doctor's consent . . . [physician-assisted suicide] is no milestone on the road to individual freedom. . . . [It] has nothing to do with the freedom of the individual and everything to do with the power of doctors.**

—Sheldon Richman, "The Fraud of Physician-Assisted Suicide," Future of Freedom Foundation, June 23, 2004. www.fff.org.

Richman is senior fellow at the Future of Freedom Foundation, author of *Tethered Citizens: Time to Repeal the Welfare State,* and editor of the *Freeman* magazine.

* Editor's Note: While the definition of a primary source can be narrowly or broadly defined, for the purposes of Compact Research, a primary source consists of: 1) results of original research presented by an organization or researcher; 2) eyewitness accounts of events, personal experience, or work experience; 3) first-person editorials offering pundits' opinions; 4) government officials presenting political plans and/or policies; 5) representatives of organizations presenting testimony or policy.

Primary Source Quotes

66 [Assisted suicide] should be allowed to take place only after all those involved are confident that the patient is not merely depressed and have had numerous opportunities to re-examine their decisions.99

—Amitai Etzioni, "No State Intrusion in End-of-Life Issues," *New Jersey Law Journal*, December 5, 2005.

Etzioni is an Israeli American sociologist, famous for his work on socioeconomics and communitarianism.

66 The misery my Mom would have suffered without that option [of physician-assisted suicide] is unthinkable. . . . To have not supported Mom in exercising that option would have been totally and unbelievably selfish.99

—Steve Harding, "Courage and Dignity: A Family's Pride," *Death with Dignity National Center*, October 14, 2005. *www.deathwithdignity.org.*

Harding's mother committed physician-assisted suicide on September 22, 2005.

66 If people around me had taken seriously . . . my cries after the accident that my life was over and I wanted to die, I might not be sitting here today, living a full, rich, though sometimes challenging life. . . . Our goal should be to eliminate the problem, not the patient.99

—Jean Swenson, "Better Dead than Disabled . . . 25 Years Later," *Human Life Alliance*, October 27, 2005. www.humanlife.org.

Swenson is a quadriplegic who obtained an MA in counseling psychology after her accident.

❝Assurances of a peaceful death when and if suffering becomes unbearable gives patients hope, comfort and peace of mind. It prevents violent, premature actions by people when facing death.❞

—Booth Gardner, "Assurances of a Peaceful Death," *Seattle Times*, April 13, 2006. http://archives.seattletimes.nwsource.com.

Gardner served as governor of Washington State from 1985 to 1993.

❝Assisting suicide is not a merciful or compassionate act. There is nothing dignified in killing yourself or assisting another in killing themselves. Assisting suicide is mere abandonment of the ill.❞

—Karen Ward, "Differentiating Assisted Suicide and Euthanasia," *North Country Gazette*, March 1, 2006. www.northcountrygazette.org.

Ward is a registered nurse with a specialty in obstetrics.

❝Better pain management, palliative care and hospice, and an increased quality of life would make this issue [of assisted suicide] a moot point. We need to work toward better life, not toward ways to end it.❞

—Richard Radtke, "A Case Against Physician-Assisted Suicide," *Journal of Disability Policy Studies*, Summer 2005.

Radtke is president of the Sea of Dreams Foundation, a nonprofit organization dedicated to helping disadvantaged individuals achieve their fullest potential and quality of life.

"I have seen close up that palliative pain management is not always 100% effective. Those who choose to opt out of this pain . . . are no less noble than those who choose to fight the pain."

—Russell Shaw, "I'm Proud to Be from the 'Death with Dignity' State of Oregon," *Huffington Post*, January 17, 2006.

Shaw is a technology and politics author, journalist, blogger, and consultant in Portland, Oregon.

....

"Doctor-assisted suicide . . . undermines trust in the patient-physician relationship."

—Kenneth Stevens, William Toffler, and Charles J. Bentz, "Physician-Assisted Suicide—Oregon—An Anomaly; Not a Harbinger," *Physicians for Compassionate Care*, August 30, 2006. www.pccef.org.

Physicians for Compassionate Care is an association of physicians and other health professionals who believe that the physician's primary task is to heal when possible, and never intentionally harm.

....

"Legalizing physician-assisted suicide . . . brings the issue out into the open and thus makes it easier to scrutinize what is actually happening and to prevent harm to the vulnerable."

—Peter Singer, "Decisions About Death," *Free Inquiry*, August/September 2005.

Singer is DeCamp Professor of Bioethics at the University Center for Human Values at Princeton University and author of *Rethinking Life and Death*.

....

66 Dutch studies . . . substantiate the suspicion that granting physicians the legal liberty to intentionally bring about the death of a patient could result in people being killed who did not ask to die. 99

—Carrie Gordon Earll, "Dutch (Holland/Netherlands) Euthanasia: The Dutch Diaster," *Focus on the Family,* September 22, 2003. www.family.org.

Earll is senior policy analyst for bioethics at Focus on the Family, and a fellow with the Center for Bioethics and Human Dignity.

66 The available data [from Oregon] demonstrate that making the option of assisted dying available, far from posing any hazard to patients or the practice of medicine, has galvanized improvements in end of life care, benefiting all terminally ill. 99

—Kathryn L. Tucker, testimony before the Senate Judiciary Committee, Subcommittee on the Constitution, Civil Rights, and Property Rights, "The Consequences of Legalized Assisted Suicide and Euthanasia," May 25, 2006. www.compassionandchoices.org.

Tucker is director of legal affairs for Compassion & Choices—an organization that supports physician-assisted suicide—and an affiliate professor of law at the University of Washington School of Law.

66 It is clear . . . that the choice is between making medically assisted dying lawful and regulated, or allowing it to continue 'underground' without any safeguards, transparency or accountability. 99

—Joel Joffe, "Death with Dignity or a License to Kill?" *Yorkshire Post,* May 12, 2006. www.ypn.co.uk.

Joffe is a retired human rights lawyer and a member of the House of Lords, the upper house of the British Parliament.

Is Physician-Assisted Suicide Ethical?

- According to *USA Today*, of Oregon's thirty thousand deaths in 2003, just forty-two were assisted-suicide cases, or 0.14 percent of the total.

- Despite support from a majority of the general public for right-to-die policies, in 2006 state legislators in California defeated a bill that would allow for physician-assisted suicide for the terminally ill.

- According to a recent Gallup poll, U.S. Catholics are more likely to support physician-assisted suicide than U.S. Protestants.

- Between 2003 and 2006, 246 terminally ill people in Oregon have chosen to end their lives by means of physician-assisted suicide.

- A 2006 Gallup poll found that some 70 percent of whites in the United States find physician-assisted suicide acceptable, as opposed to 56 percent of African Americans.

- According to the University of Washington School of Medicine, about one in five doctors receives a request for physician-assisted suicide sometime in their careers. Between 5 and 20 percent of those requests are honored.

- In a 2002 poll, the Canadian polling firm COMPAS found that some 55 percent of Canadians supported physician-assisted suicide.

Assisted Suicide on the Rise in Oregon

In October 1997 Oregon passed a state law allowing doctors to prescribe medication to patients wanting to commit suicide. Although fewer people in the state chose assisted suicide in 2004 than in 2002, the general trend has been upward since legalization.

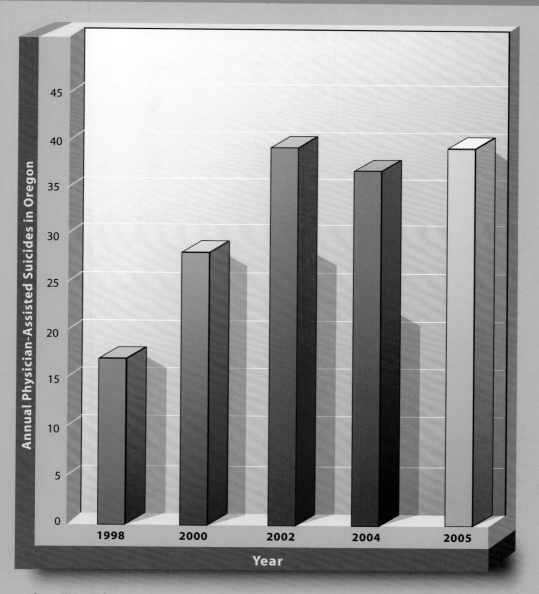

Source: Warren Richey, "High Court Takes Up Physician-Assisted Suicide," *Christian Science Monitor,* October 5, 2005.

- In order to take advantage of Oregon's Death with Dignity law, a person must first prove that he or she is a resident of the state by showing a driver's license, voter registration, and/or documentation of ownership of property in Oregon.

Support for Physician-Assisted Suicide Increasing

Since 1973 more people have supported physician-assisted suicide than not. In 2006 nearly 70 percent of Americans supported physician-assisted suicide.

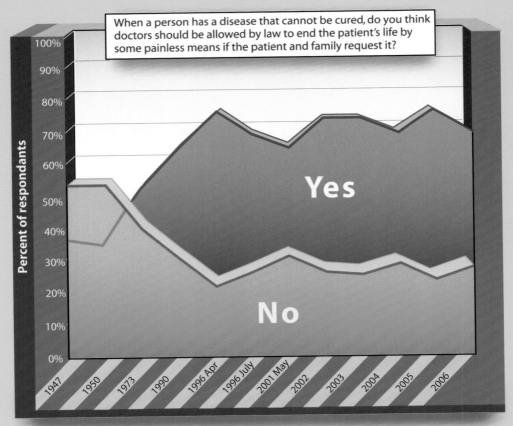

When a person has a disease that cannot be cured, do you think doctors should be allowed by law to end the patient's life by some painless means if the patient and family request it?

Source: Joseph Carroll, "Public Continues to Support Right-to-Die for Terminally Ill Patients," Gallup New Service, June 6, 2006. www.deathwithdignity.org.

How Doctors Feel About Physician-Assisted Suicide

While the majority of doctors support physician-assisted suicide, their support is less than that of the general American public. Recent polls indicate public support for PAS at almost 70 percent and doctors' support at 59 percent.

Do you think physicians should be given the right to dispense prescriptions to patients wanting to end their life?

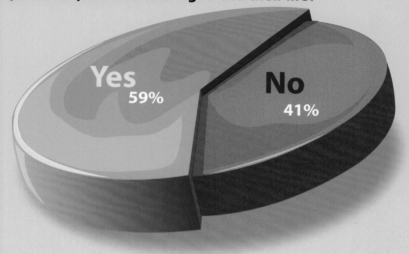

Yes 59%

No 41%

Source: HCD Research, 2005.

- Recent polls reveal that about 82 percent of politically liberal Americans support the practice of physician-assisted suicide, as compared to about 57 percent of conservatives.

- In response to challenges by the U.S. Attorney General's Office to Oregon's Death with Dignity law allowing physician-assisted suicide, in January 2006 the U.S. Supreme Court rejected the challenges and upheld Oregon's law.

Support for Physician-Assisted Suicide Varies by Race and Church Attendance

While gender does not show a significant variance in support for physician-assisted suicide, race and church attendance appear to play a role in shaping opinions on the practice. Blacks are much less likely to support physician-assisted suicide than whites. Similarly, frequent church-goers are less likely to support the practice than those who never attend church.

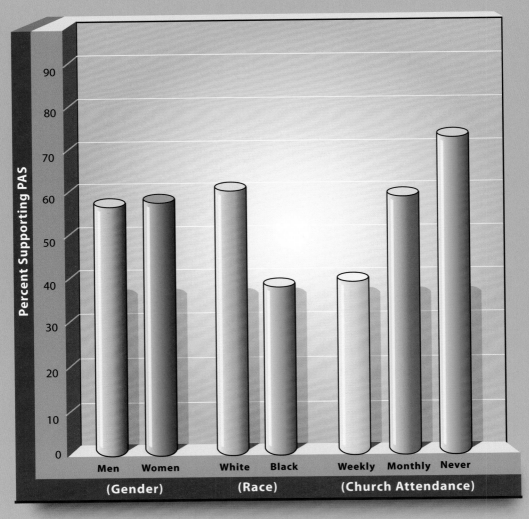

Source: Joseph Carroll, "Public Continues to Support Right-to-Die for Terminally Ill Patients," Gallup New Service, June 6, 2006. www.deathwithdignity.org.

Are Some Kinds of Genetic Testing Unethical?

"Genetic information is being generated much more quickly than our legal and social service systems can respond."

—Council for Responsible Genetics, "Genetic Discrimination." www.gene-watch.org.

A number of ethical questions surround genetic testing, more properly called genetic screening, which has been a valuable medical and scientific tool since the 1960s. The technology allows doctors and researchers to examine a sample of tissue, blood, or other specimen from a living thing and determine its genetic makeup. In terms of human beings, genetic screening is done both before birth (prenatal, or fetal) and after birth (postnatal).

Several types of each of these approaches exist. Among the best known is DNA testing performed in labs to determine if a suspect was or was not at the scene of a crime, a situation made famous by TV crime shows such as *CSI: Crime Scene Investigation.*

Another familiar kind of genetic screening of adults, carrier screening, tests prospective parents to see if they are carriers of debilitating genetic disorders. The disorders most often tested for are cystic fibrosis, Tay-Sachs disease, sickle-cell anemia, hemophilia, Huntington's disease, and neurofibromatosis. The purpose of carrier screening is to allow potential parents who do test positive for unwanted genes to make an informed decision about whether or not to have a child, since the child of two carriers of a genetic disorder has a high likelihood of being born with that disorder.

Almost no one has any ethical or moral objections to the criminal and carrier screening types of genetic testing. But some ethical gray areas do exist in the cases of some other types, among them fetal screening, also called parental diagnosis because the parents must authorize this sort of test.

The main purpose of this procedure is to diagnose birth defects in an unborn fetus. Doctors test the fetus while it is still inside the mother's womb, looking for birth defects such as Down syndrome and spina bi-fida. Based on the results, parents may choose to abort the fetus or may simply be able to prepare for the birth of a child with a disability.

The ethical questions surrounding fetal screening, as well as some other forms of genetic testing, stem not from the genetic data gathered in the procedure, but from what people do with that data. In other words, if parents, scientists, doctors, or others use the information in what society and the law see as a responsible manner, ethical objections do not usually arise. By contrast, a number of people perceive various potential ways that this technology can be abused.

Fears of Eugenics

Some of these possible abuses of genetic screening fall under the general heading of eugenics. Noted Princeton University scientist Lee M. Silver describes the popular notion of eugenics this way:

> In its original connotation, eugenics referred to the idea that a society might be able to improve its gene pool by exerting control over the breeding practices of its citizens. In America, early twentieth-century attempts to put this idea into practice brought about the forced sterilization of people deemed genetically inferior because of (supposed) reduced intelligence, minor physical disabilities, or possession of a (supposed) criminal character. . . . Later, Nazi Germany used an even more drastic approach in its attempt to eliminate—in a single generation—those who carried undesirable genes.[25]

No one today is accusing scientists and doctors of perpetrating forced sterilizations and mass murder. However, some concerned individuals and groups worry that testing the genes of unborn children will allow parents and others to manipulate fetuses in the womb, thereby interfering with the natural process of childbirth. Such manipulation is seen by many as undesirable and wrong.

In the United States, for example, genetic screening for disabilities has become common, with parents frequently choosing to abort disabled children rather than give birth to them. Says George Neumayr, editor of *American Spectator* magazine, "The vast majority of unborn children prenatally diagnosed as disabled are killed."[26] According to Neumayr, an estimated 80 percent of babies prenatally diagnosed with Down syndrome are aborted. He worries that this trend of aborting disabled babies will lead to a society in which:

> Parents who abort their disabled children won't be asked to justify their decision. Rather, it is the parents with disabled children who must justify themselves to a society that tacitly asks: Why did you bring into the world a child you knew was disabled or might become disabled?[27]

Another use of genetic screening is to detect the gender of an unborn baby. Some parents want to know their child's gender out of curiosity and/or to allow them to plan what clothes and toys to buy in advance of the birth. Other parents, however, can and often do use this information to select babies' genders. Science writer Catherine Baker explains: "In some countries in which the culture values boys more than girls, ultrasound and [genetic screening] are used mainly to check the sex of the fetus. If the fetus is a girl, it is [often] aborted."[28]

If a baby's gender can be chosen in such a manner, some critics of genetic screening say, parents might also be able to select other traits for their babies in advance of birth, such as eye color, hair color, or even skin color. Though the technology to make so-called designer children easily and accurately is still in its infancy, many scientists

> " Some concerned individuals and groups worry that testing the genes of unborn children will allow parents and others to manipulate fetuses in the womb. "

say that it is only a matter of time before that technology is perfected. The Human Genetics Commission, a biomedical ethics think tank that advises the British government, summarizes the chief objections voiced by those who see this as a form of eugenics: "Some feel that in 'designing' babies, society is no longer valuing children for who they are, but rather for what they are, making them into consumer items, with embryos or fetuses being discarded when they are not suitable."[29]

Journalist Stephen Pinker points out that other genetically designed products have been subject to considerable social criticism, and worries about how designer babies might be received. "Many people are repelled by genetically modified foods even though they have never been shown to be unsafe or harmful to the environment," he says. "If people are repulsed by genetically modified soybeans, would they really welcome genetically modified children?"[30]

Religious Arguments Against Genetic Screening

In addition to those who worry that genetic screening is encouraging a modern upsurge of eugenics, a number of individuals and groups harbor religious objections to certain ways the technology is used. For instance, the Catholic Church accepts genetic testing if the sole goals of the procedure are to inform the parents of their unborn child's condition and to set in motion any therapies or cures that might be possible. However, the church does not support such procedures when they are used to promote practices such as eugenics and abortion, both of which church leaders heartily condemn. As the late Pope John Paul II put it:

> It not infrequently happens that these techniques are used . . . to prevent the birth of children affected by various types of anomalies. Such an attitude is shameful and utterly reprehensible, since it presumes to measure the value of a human life only within the parameters of "normality" and physical well-being.[31]

Another religious objection to genetic testing focuses more on God and his supposed plans for Earth and humanity than on the physical well-being of the people and fetuses involved. Some critics believe that humans should not be interfering with God's creation. Such religious objections to genetic screening are by no means limited to the United States. According to science writer Karina Monteiro;

> Mostly motivated by religion, some parts of the world don't accept genetic testing, having the thought and reasoning that a child is a gift and it should be accepted no matter what is wrong with it. Some religions even believe that having a child with a defect is a spiritual and beautiful thing.[32]

Discrimination and Privacy Issues

Still another objection to genetic screening concerns genetic tests done on living humans in which the information revealed is used to violate a person's rights, dignity, or privacy. One common worry, for instance, is that if people learn that a certain individual has "inferior" genes, they will discriminate against him or her in various ways. The person might be discouraged from reproducing by family and friends; or someone might suffer racial or ethnic discrimination if it is revealed that he or she carries a gene closely associated with Jews, blacks, or members of other minorities.

Cited even more frequently in recent years is potential discrimination by employers against employees or insurance companies against clients whose genetic tests have revealed that they have—or might in the future have—serious health problems. Both employers and insurers are sometimes reluctant to continue dealing with a person who might end up costing them what they see as too much money. Patrick Dixon, chairman of Global Change (a company that analyses social and economic trends world wide), explains how genetic testing might affect some people. He says, "The fear is that gene screening for insurance will mean that some individuals with gene problems will become uninsurable for life or health coverage and will form a

> " One common worry . . . is that if people learn that a certain individual has "inferior" genes, they will discriminate against him or her in various ways. "

genetic underclass, unable to get a house mortgage for example."[33] The Council for Responsible Genetics, a nonprofit organization based in Cambridge, Massachusetts, believes it would be unfair to make employment or insurance decisions based on genetic characteristics acquired at birth. It argues, "Whereas individuals can exercise choices about whether to smoke, how much exercise they get, and how much fat is in their diets, they cannot change the contents of their genes."[34]

In a similar vein, some people worry that the results of their genetic tests will fall into the hands of the police and other law enforcement organizations. The fear is that such groups might use such information in illegal or unethical ways. They might coerce a person into confessing to crimes he or she did not commit, for example, or into unfairly incriminating someone else. To combat such discrimination, some states, along with some foreign countries, have begun to pass laws barring employers, insurance companies, and police organizations from misusing people's genetic information. Comprehensive legislation is still years away in most places, however. In the meantime, it is up to each individual to exercise caution when having any sort of genetic screening done by making sure that the clinic or lab doing the tests keeps the results private.

In fact, resolution of such privacy issues may actually be the key to the future success or failure of some forms of genetic screening. It is possible, asserts Arthur Caplan, director of the Center for Bioethics at the University of Pennsylvania, that in years to come a majority of people will choose to avoid such screening for fear that the results will fall into the wrong hands. "Without some form of better privacy protection, genetic testing is not going to flourish," Caplan says. Without such protection, he adds, "genetic testing is not going to go anywhere because it's going to founder on the rock of privacy."[35]

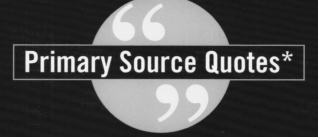

Are Some Kinds of Genetic Testing Unethical?

> **Genetic engineering . . . [will one day allow you to] improve the genetic makeup of your children: to prevent them from getting genetic diseases, to prolong their lifespan. . . . You should have such rights just as you have the right to vaccinate your children.**

—Alex Epstein, "Cloning Is Moral," *Ayn Rand Institute*, February 13, 2004. www.aynrand.org.

Epstein is a writer for the Ayn Rand Institute, an organization dedicated to promoting the principles of individual rights.

> **Allowing genetic 'enhancements' in humans would unleash a powerful new eugenics, and could lead to unacceptable forms of genetic discrimination and inequality.**

—Andrew Kimbrell, "Cloning: A Risk to Women?" testimony before the Senate Committee on Commerce, Science, and Transportation, Subcommitte on Science, Technology, and Space, March 27, 2003. http://commerce.senate.gov.

Kimbrell is executive director of the International Center for Technology Assessment.

* Editor's Note: While the definition of a primary source can be narrowly or broadly defined, for the purposes of Compact Research, a primary source consists of: 1) results of original research presented by an organization or researcher; 2) eyewitness accounts of events, personal experience, or work experience; 3) first-person editorials offering pundits' opinions; 4) government officials presenting political plans and/or policies; 5) representatives of organizations presenting testimony or policy.

66 **Dramatic improvements in the lives of our children are well within our reach, and require no manipulation of inheritable genes.** 99

—Center for Genetics and Society, "Perspectives: Children's and Family Advocates," May 30, 2003. www.genetics-and-society.org.

The Center for Genetics and Society is a nonprofit organization working to encourage responsible uses of new human genetic and reproductive technologies.

66 **[The ability to select genetic traits for babies] would benefit the rich far more than the poor. They would take the gap . . . that currently divides . . . our society . . . and write that division into our very biology.** 99

—Bill McKibben, "Designer Genes," *Orion*, May/June 2003. www.orionsociety.org.

McKibben is the author of *The End of Nature* and *Enough: Staying Human in an Engineered Age*.

66 **[Genetic screening] means . . . that thousands of parents who are at known risk of passing on terrible disabilities and diseases will now be able to have only healthy babies. This is the best news I have heard for years.** 99

—Minette Marrin, "Scientists Playing God? We Should Rejoice," *TimesOnline*, June 25, 2006. www.timesonline.co.uk.

Marrin is a journalist, broadcaster, and fiction writer.

66 **Disability is a natural part of the human experience. . . . Disability need not be seen as a tragedy to be avoided [through genetic testing].** 99

—Andrew J. Imparato, "Prenatal Genetic Testing Technology," testimony before the Senate Committee on Commerce, Science, and Transportation, Subcommittee on Science, Technology, and Space, November 17, 2004. http://commerce.senate.gov.

Imparato is president of the American Association of People with Disabilities.

❝I was . . . appalled to learn that doctors plan to create designer babies free from autism. . . . [My autistic son] Danny is the best thing that has ever happened to me and the idea that we might have somehow been 'better off' if he had never been born is intolerable.❞

—Virginia Bovell, "We Don't Need to Wipe Out Autism . . . We Need to Care More," *Daily Mail*, June 19, 2006. www.dailymail.co.uk.

Bovell is the mother of an eleven-year-old boy with autism.

❝[Genetic testing] may cause irreparable damage in the parent child bond . . . [because of] how they view those who have had 'abnormal testing' but are completely normal human beings.❞

—John Bruchalski, "Prenatal Genetic Testing Technology," testimony before the Senate Committee on Commerce, Science, and Transportation Subcommittee on Science, Technology, and Space, November 17, 2004. http://commerce.senate.gov.

Bruchalski is a physician who has been in practice since 1987.

❝[Genetic] tests could improve hiring decisions. . . . For example, if a small number of individuals have a genetic tendency to get sick from a certain toxin in the workplace, then screening these individuals can protect the employer from an expensive lawsuit.❞

—Asher Meir, "Genetic Testing in the Workplace," Business Ethics Center of Jerusalem, October 14, 2005. www.besr.org.

Meir is research director of the Business Ethics Center of Jerusalem, an organization that works to encourage and promote a high standard of business integrity and economic honesty.

66 **Genetic testing is clearly harmful if the information is used to deny jobs or insurance, or if it leads to other forms of discrimination.** 99

—United Cerebral Palsy and the Arc of the United States, statement regarding Request for Public Comment on Genetic Discrimination, September 17, 2004. www.thearc.org.

United Cerebral Palsy is a national organization committed to enhancing the lives of people with disabilities. The Arc of the United States is the national organization for people with mental retardation and their families.

66 **Genetic tests . . . [may] be misleading. . . . At worst, they may also be harmful to health. . . . Genes are generally poor predictors of common diseases and this approach is likely to lead to many people receiving unnecessary and potentially harmful treatment.** 99

—Helen M. Wallace, "Misleading Marketing of Genetic Tests," *Council for Responsible Genetics*, March/April 2005. www. gene-watch.org.

Wallace is deputy director of GeneWatch UK, an organization that aims to ensure genetic technologies are used in the public interest.

66 **I decided not to undergo testing [for a possible genetic predisposition to breast cancer] for fear of potential consequences to my daughter. . . . If I test positive, my daughter might be obligated to disclose the presence of a genetic mutation and . . . she might suffer future discrimination in health insurance and employment as a consequence.** 99

—Carolina Hinestrosa, testimony before the Secretary's Advisory Committee on Genetics, Health, and Society, National Institutes of Health, October 18-19, 2004. www4.od.nih.gov.

Hinestosa is a two-time breast cancer survivor and executive vice president of the National Breast Cancer Coalition.

Facts and Illustrations

Are Some Kinds of Genetic Testing Unethical?

- According to a 2004 survey conducted by the Genetic Public Policy Center, 35 percent of Americans feel that genetic testing is like "playing God."

- Genetic testing used to identify the birth father of a child can have accuracy rates as high as 99.99 percent.

- Fewer than half of the United States—twenty-three to be exact—have laws protecting the privacy of genetic information.

- Twenty-one states have enacted laws protecting citizens from discrimination in employment based on the results of genetic screening.

- According to the directors of the Human Genome Project, some 950 genetic tests can now be conducted in modern labs and many more are presently in development.

- The U.S. Department of Energy Office of Science estimates that most genetic tests cost between two hundred and three thousand dollars.

- As of March 2006 State and federal databases held genetic screening profiles of 2.9 million people which provided useful leads in approximately 32,000 criminal investigations.

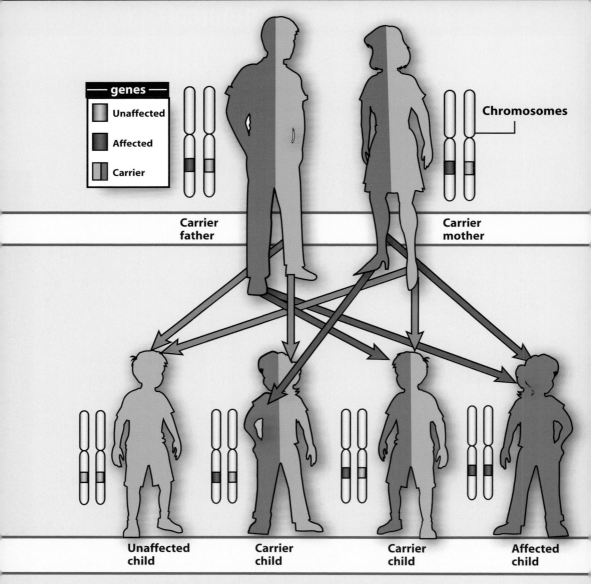

How a Genetic Condition Is Passed On

This illustration shows how a father and mother can pass on a gene that can cause a disease such as cancer. In this case, to get the disease a person must receive the affected gene from both the mother and father. Of the four children, only one received the affected gene from both parents and will consequently develop the disease. Two of the children have one affected gene and will be carriers. In this way, genetic screening can be used by a couple to determine the likelihood of passing on a disease to their children. This can help people in making reproductive decisions.

genes

Unaffected

Affected

Carrier

Chromosomes

Carrier
father

Carrier
mother

Unaffected
child

Carrier
child

Carrier
child

Affected
child

Source: National Library of Medicine, "Inheritance Patterns," 2006. http://ghr.nlm.nih.gov.

- The U.S. Department of Health and Human Services says that more than four thousand diseases are passed via genes within families. Fewer than a quarter of these diseases have reliable genetic tests.

- Scientists estimate that 5 to 10 percent of all cancers are genetic, and therefore can potentially be predicted through genetic testing.

- U.S. federal agencies are currently prohibited from discriminating against people on the basis of the results of genetic tests.

Social Concerns About Genetic Testing

This survey indicates that the majority of Americans are concerned about the social implications of genetic testing. Over 80 percent are concerned that genetic screening for disibilites stigmatizes the disabled and will lead to discrimination. Over two-thirds worry that the ability to choose the sex of a baby will lead to gender imbalance.

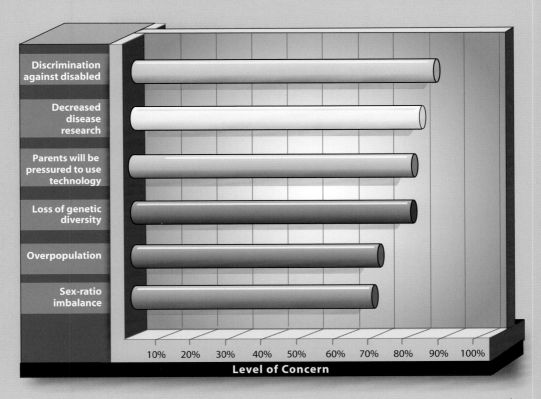

Source: Genetics and Public Policy Center, 2004.

Reproductive Genetic Testing and "Designer Children"

The ability to control human reproduction will lead to treating children like products.

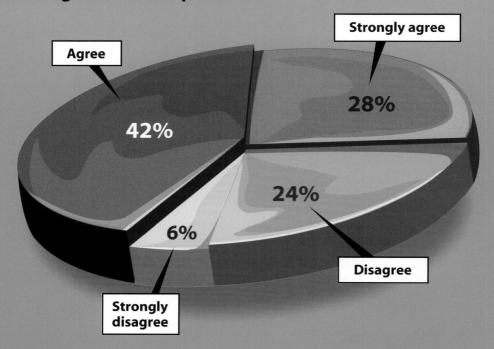

Seventy percent of Americans believe that reproductive genetic testing will lead to parents selecting children like they would products. Critics of genetic screening argue that designing children is unethical and will increase abortion rates as fetuses with undesirable traits will be terminated.

Source: Genetics and Public Policy Center, 2004.

Should Human Embryos Be Used in Stem Cell Research?

Should Human Embryos Be Used in Stem Cell Research?

> **Should we . . . permit destructive embryonic stem cell research because of its remarkable potential benefits? Or should we . . . prohibit destructive embryonic stem cell research because it violates respect for . . . the very beginnings of a possible human life?**

—Maurice Rickard, "Key Ethical Issues in Embryonic Stem Cell Research," *Current Issues Brief*, no. 5, November 12, 2002.

It is widely recognized that among the more outstanding scientific achievements of the last decades of the twentieth century was the discovery and initial understanding of human embryonic stem cells. Many people—scientists and nonscientists alike—view ongoing stem cell research as a sort of medical miracle that holds almost unlimited promise for future generations of human beings. In the words of Thomas B. Okarma, a former physician at the Stanford University School of Medicine, "The potential of these cells is . . . to broaden the definition of medical therapy from simply halting the progression of . . . disease to include restoration of lost organ function."[36]

An Enormous Potential

The main reason embryonic stem cells, or ES cells, offer hope for restoring lost or damaged organs is that these cells possess some unusual properties that most other body cells lack. First, human ES cells are undifferentiated, or unspecialized, cells. In other words, they are cells that have not yet received specific instructions to become specific kinds of cells, such as those making up a person's bones, skin, heart, or brain. Second, ES cells are easily grown in large, usable quantities. "They have the ability to self-renew," one expert explains, "which means that they are theoretically immortal and can continue to divide forever if provided with enough nutrients."[37]

These unique qualities provide researchers with the potential of growing ES cells into almost any kind of tissue that doctors and patients might need, including skin tissues or even entire organs such as livers or kidneys. These tissues or organs could then be used to replace or repair damaged or diseased versions, opening up new vistas in organ transplant operations. In the past, a great deal of research has been done on using animal organs for human transplants. That approach still shows some degree of promise. However, its major inherent drawback is that animal organs are more often than not rejected by the human immune system. In the case of tissues and organs grown from ES cells, in contrast, the patient will receive a version of his or her own cells. So the match will be genetically perfect and no rejection will occur.

> " Researchers say that . . . burn victims will be able to receive healthy new skin grown from tiny samples of their own tissues. "

Virtually all members of the scientific and medical communities agree that the potential benefits of transplanting tissues and organs the body will readily accept rather than reject are nothing less than enormous. Researchers say that a host of beneficial transplants will be possible using human ES cells. For example, burn victims will be able to receive healthy new skin grown from tiny samples of their own tissues; people with spinal cord injuries will have their spines repaired; and hearts, lungs, bladders, and other organs will be literally made to order for specific patients, saving or extending their lives. In addition, says one expert, "Mastery of the stem cell might lead to . . . ways to eliminate many genetic diseases through DNA engineering, while extending the human life span."[38]

Federal Funding for ES Cell Research

However promising embryonic stem cells may be to scientists, doctors, and patients, some people voice ethical concerns about their use. The primary concern is that ES cell research involves the creation and destruction of human embryos, which, in the eyes of the critics, are potential human beings. According to this view, when a scientist manipulates an ES cell, causing it to begin replicating itself over and over again, he or she destroys its ability to grow into a viable human fetus. Thus, manipulating stem cells this way is a form of murder.

> **Research into the regenerative possibilities of human ES cells continues at an increasing pace in a number of foreign nations.**

Among the high-profile people who have taken this right-to-life position on human ES cells is President George W. Bush. During his first year in office he came under considerable pressure from the scientific and medical communities to approve federal funding for ES cell research. However, the president also felt pressure from those who are against such research, including evangelical Christians and other conservatives. In an attempt to satisfy both sides while staying true to his own religious and ethical beliefs, in 2001 he approved federal funding for a limited number of ES cell lines (groups of cells, each grown from a single master cell). These lines had already been created and used for replication in various labs, so the proposed funding would not involve the creation and destruction of any new ES cells. Says Bush, "This policy has allowed research to go forward and has allowed America to continue to lead the world in embryonic stem cell research without encouraging the further destruction of living human embryos."[39]

The problem with Bush's approach, according to many scientists and doctors, was that the lines of ES cells he approved have severe limitations for research. According to this view, they are too old. More specifically, they were originally cultured using methods that are now outdated, and as a result they are less robust and viable than fresher stem cells. "They can't do what the newer cell lines can do," argues Curt Civin, a cancer researcher at Johns Hopkins Medical School. "We're working with version 1.0," he adds. "I'd like version 3.3."[40]

Meanwhile, the president's denial of federal funding for ES cell lines beyond those he approved has no bearing on what privately funded labs do, nor on ES cell research in other countries. In fact research into the regenerative possibilities of human ES cells continues at an

Library
Academy of the Holy Cross
4920 Strathmore Avenue
Kensington, MD 20895

increasing pace in a number of foreign nations. This worries many experts in the United States, who fear that American labs, universities, and companies are losing the lead in developing this new technology. In addition, experts worry that because it is not federally approved, the research being conducted in the United States may not be open to public scrutiny. As journalist Gregg Easterbrook explains, "Congress has created the preposterous situation in which most stem cell research is not being done by publicly funded scientists who must pass multiple levels of peer review."[41]

Human Rights: The Living Versus the Unborn

Fueling the arguments on both sides of the debate about government funding for ES cell research are strong opposing opinions about whether the ethical concerns of one segment of the population should outweigh the needs of suffering patients. All involved in the debate acknowledge that the choices involved are difficult. This is partly because scientists, doctors, and policy makers find themselves confronting the needs and rights of what some people see as two groups of living beings. On one hand are the existing humans who struggle with various medical conditions and who might benefit from ES cell research; on the other are the potential humans who may someday grow from the embryos that scientists want to use in such research. Some bioethicists say that it is likely that over time the needs of already living people will supercede those of people yet unborn.

> A number of bioethicists and concerned citizens think that the unborn have rights ... and meddling with human embryos in any way abridges these rights.

Harvard University president Lawrence H. Summers agrees. He says, "The life-and-death medical needs of countless suffering children and adults justifies moving forward with [embryonic stem cell] research."[42]

In contrast, a number of bioethicists and concerned citizens think that the unborn have rights too. According to this view, these rights must be protected at all costs, and meddling with human embryos in any way abridges these rights. Hannah M. Vick, of the influential public policy organization Concerned Women for America, concisely sums up this view, saying:

> Human embryos are not simply tissue to be researched. The underlying utilitarian belief that some humans need to be sacrificed for the betterment of others is morally and ethically wrong. . . . Human beings, at any stage of development, should not be drafted for research without their permission—no matter what the supposed justification.[43]

Are Adult Stem Cells an Ethical Alternative?

Those who oppose research using human ES cells often promote the idea of using what they claim is a perfectly viable alternative to embryonic stem cells, namely adult stem cells. Adult stem cells are undifferentiated cells found in several of the body's organs. Although some uncertainty remains, most scientists think that the natural purpose of these cells, which exist in far smaller numbers than differentiated cells in these organs, is to aid in tissue regeneration after an injury. Australian senator Brian Harradine is an advocate of adult stem cells. He says, "There are already adult stem cell cures that do not have any of the problems of . . . destroying human embryos." According to Harradine, critics imply that failing to allow embryonic stem cell research will halt valuable research that may cure many diseases, but this is simply not true. He maintains, "No cures have resulted so far from embryonic stem cell research and there are serious doubts they will."[44] The Stem Cell Research Foundation disagrees. "Many people ask why embryonic stem cells are needed when adult bodies also produce stem cells," asks the foundation. "The answer is that they are not the same. . . . While it is possible that scientists may someday be able to accomplish the same goals with adult cells as embryonic ones, that day could be many years in the future."[45]

One drawback of adult stem cells is that they are difficult to grow and multiply in a lab. However, some hope for the use of these cells does exist, as several researchers have reported initial successes in increasing their numbers and viability. Late in 2005, for instance, Harvey Lodish, a professor and medical researcher at MIT, found a way to force adult stem cells to multiply much faster than was possible in the past. Whether this technology will lead to the production of replacement organs made from adult stem cells remains to be seen, but Lodish and others view it as at least an important first step toward that goal.

Finding an Ethical Compromise

Whatever the future medical potential of adult stem cells may be, they remain one of the key issues in the present debate over the morality of using embryonic stem cells. In spite of the ethical arguments against ES cells and for adult stem cells, however, the vast majority of scientists feel that it is unwise to pursue one kind of stem cell at the expense of the other. "There are camps for adult stems cells and embryonic stem cells," states Douglas Melton of the Harvard Stem Cell Institute in Cambridge, Massachusetts. "But these camps exist only in the political arena. There is no disagreement among scientists over the need to aggressively pursue both in order to solve important medical problems."[46]

Indeed, each year more and more scientists, physicians, politicians, and ordinary citizens come to appreciate the potential benefits of all stem cell research, especially that involving ES cells. In fact, the huge medical potential of embryonic stem cells makes it no longer a matter of if these cells will be widely used. As Arthur Caplan of the Center for Bioethics at the University of Pennsylvania points out, "The value of embryonic stem cell research is simply too great to permit a policy stance of inaction to be the response that our government and other governments around the world offer to this enormously promising domain of inquiry."[47]

> **The huge medical potential of embryonic stem cells makes it no longer a matter of if these cells will be widely used.**

It therefore becomes more a matter of how embryonic stem cells will be used. Will they be employed in experiments approved and funded by the U.S. government? Or will such approval and funding be withheld because of a lack of public consensus about the morality of experiments involving ES cells? In this regard, a number of experts stress the importance of achieving some sort of balance between scientific needs and progress in stem cell research and ethical concerns about that research. As Santa Clara University scholar Margaret R. McLean puts it:

> It is important that we do not prematurely or unwittingly slam the door on scientific advances [in the area of stem cells]. . . . At the same time, it is imperative that . . . we . . . concern ourselves with the shaping of a just future. . . . If we wisely engage in shaping the future [of stem cell research], we will create a world few of us ever imagined.[48]

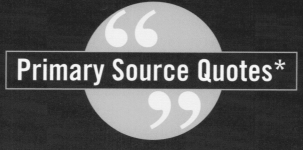

Primary Source Quotes*

Should Human Embryos Be Used in Stem Cell Research?

66 Embryonic stem cells come from human embryos that are destroyed for their cells. Each of these human embryos is a unique life with inherent dignity and matchless value. . . . Not spare parts. 99

—George W. Bush, "President Discusses Stem Cell Research Policy," July 19, 2006. www.whitehouse.gov.

Bush is the forty-third president of the United States.

66 Yes, these [embryonic stem] cells could theoretically have the potential . . . to develop into human beings. . . . But they are not, in and of themselves, human beings. They have no fingers and toes, no brain or spinal cord. They have no thoughts, no fears. 99

—Ron Reagan Jr., *PBS Online NewsHour*, July 27, 2004. www.pbs.org.

Reagan Jr. is a political commentator and son of late former U.S. president Ronald Reagan.

* Editor's Note: While the definition of a primary source can be narrowly or broadly defined, for the purposes of Compact Research, a primary source consists of: 1) results of original research presented by an organization or researcher; 2) eyewitness accounts of events, personal experience, or work experience; 3) first-person editorials offering pundits' opinions; 4) government officials presenting political plans and/or policies; 5) representatives of organizations presenting testimony or policy.

❝The early human embryo . . . [is] a human life deserving moral respect. . . . Stem cell research that requires destroying human embryos is unethical.❞

—Richard M. Doerflinger, testimony before the Commonwealth of Virginia Joint Subcommittee Studying Medical, Ethical, and Scientific Issues Relating to Stem Cell Research, November 15, 2005. www.stemcellresearch.org.

Doerflinger is deputy director of the Secretariat for Pro-Life Activities at the U.S. Conference of Catholic Bishops.

❝Surely it is . . . permissible for some embryos to die for the values of health, wellbeing and longevity [that might be achieved through embryonic stem cell research].❞

—Julian Savulescu, "Recent Advances in Stem Cell Science and Therapies," *Australian Academy of Science*, May 6, 2005. www.science.org.

Savulescu is Uehiro Chair in practical ethics at the University of Oxford, Australia. He is also head of the Melbourne-Oxford Stem Cell Collaboration, devoted to examining the ethical implications of cloning and embryonic stem cell research.

❝I'll never walk again. I don't believe that stem-cell therapies will be developed in my lifetime. . . . But the thought of young people who have a real chance for recovery, their hopes stymied by a simple-minded attempt to stop [embryonic stem cell research] . . . is simply too much for me to bear.❞

—Martin Kace, "A Few Facts About My Existence," *Beliefnet*, August 4, 2006. www.beliefnet.com.

Kace is paralyzed from the chest down.

66 [Researchers] will have greater impact by focusing on animal embryonic stem-cell research and adult stem-cell research, which do not require . . . [the] moral and ethical trespasses [that embryonic stem cell research does]. 99

—James L. Sherley, "Crossing Line on Cloning," *Boston Globe*, June 12, 2006. www.boston.com.

Sherley is a stem cell biologist at the Massachusetts Institute of Technology.

66 We know too little to leap to grand conclusions about which cells and which methods will ultimately prove useful. . . . [We] should be encouraging every possible line of research. Only then can we be sure that the treatments for which so many people are desperate will arrive. 99

—*New Scientist*, "Great Expectations: Embryonic Stem Cells Could Work Wonders—If We Knew How to Get Them," May 28, 2005.

New Scientist magazine reports on science and technology news from around the world.

66 In vitro fertilization [results in excess embryos]. . . . Given the reality that most, if not all, of these excess embryos will be discarded—we believe that it is morally tolerable to use existing embryos for stem cell research purposes. 99

—United Methodist Church, "Ethics of Embryonic Stem Cell Research," 2004. http://archives.umc.org.

The United Methodist Church was founded in 1968.

> 66 **Regardless of the numbers of embryos [left over from in vitro fertilization and] available for research, dissecting tiny humans for their cells is unethical and immoral.** 99

—Carrie Gordon Earll, "Frequently Asked Questions: Stem Cell Research," *Focus on the Family*, December 10, 2004. www.family.org.

Earll is the senior policy analyst for bioethics at Focus on the Family and a fellow with the Center for Bioethics and Human Dignity.

> 66 **Embryonic stem cells are key to the increasingly promising area of regenerative medicine, which could profoundly improve our ability to prevent and cure disease. . . . More human embryonic stem cells . . . [should] be readily available to scientists.** 99

—Juvenile Diabetes Research Foundation International, "Embryonic Stem Cells," September 2003. www.jdrf.org.

The Juvenile Diabetes Research Foundation works to find a cure for diabetes through the support of research.

> 66 **Given the immense benefits that we might derive from embryonic stem cell research, including the development or therapies that could ameliorate or eliminate many debilitating and disabling illnesses and injuries . . . support of such research . . . is of paramount importance.** 99

—Ronald A. Lindsay, "Stem Cell Research: An Approach to Bioethics Based on Scientific Naturalism," *Center for Inquiry*, July 26, 2006. www.centerforinquiry.net.

Lindsay is legal director for the Center for Inquiry, an organization that supports reason- and science-based inquiry.

❝The problem with . . . [embryonic stem cell research is that] today we kill embryos to cure disabling conditions; tomorrow we may be tempted to kill other 'marginal' humans . . . to spare their families or free funds for those thought more deserving.❞

—Stephen L. Mikochik, "Moral Equivalent of a Parkinson's Patient?" *Washington Times*, August 20, 2006. www.washington times.com.

Stephen L. Mikochik is a professor of constitutional law at Temple University, Philadelphia, and was formerly an expert on disability law in the Civil Rights Division of the U.S. Department of Justice.

....

❝[There are] serious, inherent potential problems with . . . embryonic stem cell research, including but not limited to: exploitation, fraud, and coercion.❞

—Mark Souder, opening statement to the House Committee on Government Reform, Subcommittee on Criminal Justice, Drug Policy, and Human Resources, "Human Cloning and Embryonic Stem Cell Research After Seoul: Examining Exploition, Fraud, and Ethical Problems in the Research," March 7, 2006, 109th cong., 2nd session. http://reform.house.gov.

Souder is a Republican congressman from Indiana.

....

❝[Stem cell] research offers the potential to eliminate diseases and literally save millions of lives . . . it's time to act on what we've learned.❞

—Michael J. Fox, testimony before the Senate subcommittee on Labor, Health and Human Services and Education, September 14, 2000.

Fox, a popular television and film actor, was diagnosed with Parkinson's disease in 1991. Since revealing his condition to the pubic in 1998, he has been a vocal advocate for Parkinson's and stem cell research and funding.

....

Facts and Illustrations

Should Human Embryos Be Used in Stem Cell Research?

- Human embryonic stem cell research began in 1998 when a group led by Dr. James Thompson at the University of Wisconsin developed a technique to isolate and grow the cells.

- Some 220 kinds of stem cells exist in the human body.

- In 2002 Australia's Parliament authorized the use of new human stem cell lines for research in that country.

- In December 2002 the British government approved the equivalent of $94 million for stem cell research, making British efforts in this area among the best funded in the world.

- In 2003 a RAND Corporation study found that about four hundred thousand human embryos were stored in U.S. labs, clinics, and other medical and scientific facilities.

- California's Proposition 71, which called for state funding of stem cell research, passed in November 2004 by a margin of 59 to 41 percent.

- New Jersey became the second state (after California) to permit embryonic stem cell research.

How Stem Cells Are Created

This illustration shows how specific types of cells, such as blood or muscle cells, can be reproduced from a human embryo. These cells can then be used to potentially cure sick and diseased people. However, many argue that the human embryo used in stem cell creation represents a life and to destroy the embryo even for the benefit of others is unethical.

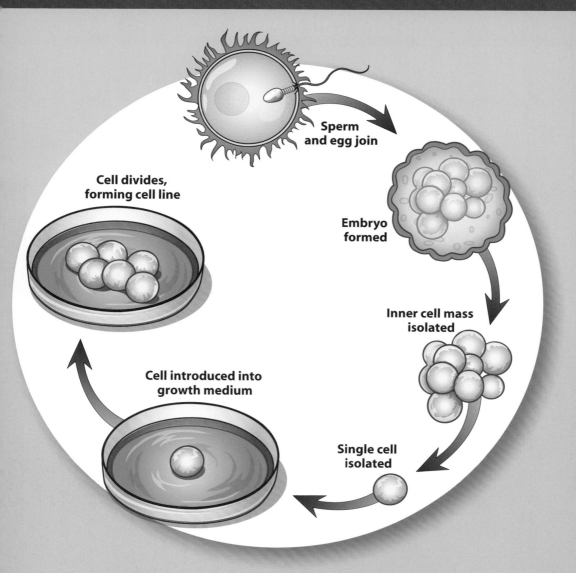

Sperm and egg join

Cell divides, forming cell line

Embryo formed

Inner cell mass isolated

Cell introduced into growth medium

Single cell isolated

Source: University of Utah, Genetic Learning Center, 2006. www.learn.genetics.utah.edu.

The Benefits of Stem Cells

Although stem cell research creates many ethical issues, it also yields important practical benefits. In addition to supporting further advancement in genetic research and drug development, stem cells have the potential to cure people with cancer and other terminal diseases.

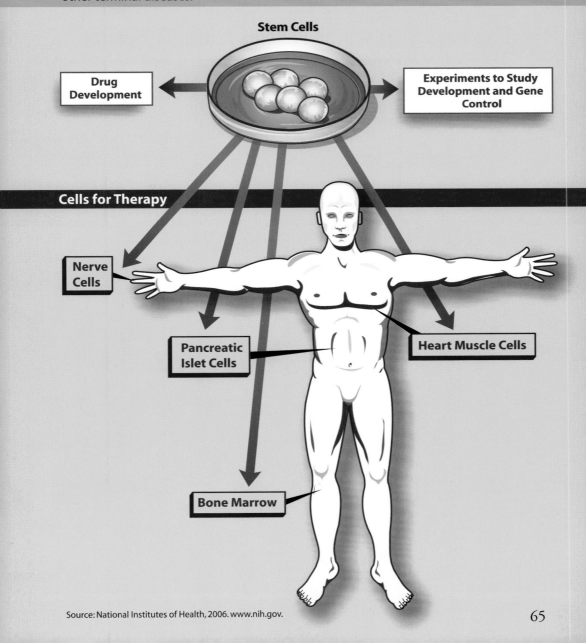

Source: National Institutes of Health, 2006. www.nih.gov.

- Stem cell research has produced seventy-two cures and treatments.

- In March 2005 a team of German scientists reported that they had grown mouse liver, muscle, and pancreas cells from stem cells taken from mouse testicles.

Stem Cell Research Policies Around the Globe

This map shows government policies on human embryonic stem cell research. The countries in blue, representing nearly half of the world population, permit embryonic stem cell research and therapeutic cloning. The countries in red allow stem cell research but only with donated embryos from fertility clinics. The countries in yellow, including the United States, Italy, and Germany, do not allow human embryonic research, have restrictive laws, or have no established policies.

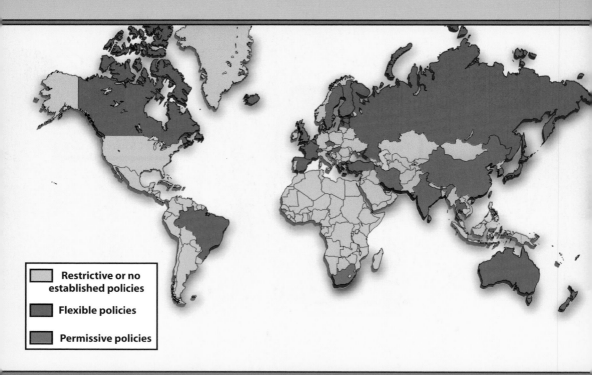

Restrictive or no established policies

Flexible policies

Permissive policies

Source: University of Minnesota Medical School, 2006. www.mbbnet.com.

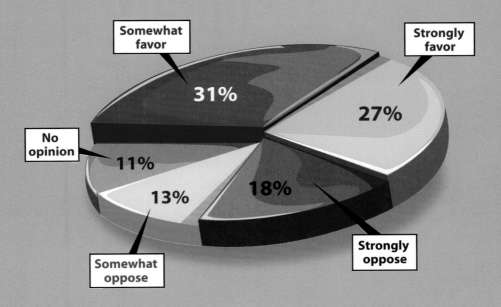

Majority of Americans Support the Use of Human Embryos for Stem Cells

On the whole, how much do you favor or oppose medical research that uses stem cells from human embryos—do you strongly favor, somewhat favor, somewhat oppose, or strongly oppose this?

Somewhat favor — 31%

Strongly favor — 27%

No opinion — 11%

13% — Somewhat oppose

18% — Strongly oppose

Although U.S. law prohibits the use of human embryos for stem cell research, the majority of Americans support this type of medical research. According to the 2005 survey 58 percent of Americans favor medical research that uses stem cells from human embryos.

Source: Virginia Commonwealth University, 2005.

- By late 2006 only twenty-one of the initial seventy-two embryonic stem cell lines authorized by President Bush in 2001 were still usable.

Should Human Cloning Be Banned?

Should Human Cloning Be Banned?

> 66 **The debate about human cloning is a debate over nothing less than what it means to be human.** 99

—Patrick Stephens, "Cloning: Towards a New Conception of Humanity?" Objectivist Center. www.objectivistcenter.org.

Cloning, in particular the possible cloning of human beings, is presently one of the most controversial and widely debated areas of biomedical ethics. Biologically speaking, a clone is the offspring of any living thing that reproduces by asexual means. In other words, a single parent, acting as the genetic donor, passes on its DNA (the complex chemical containing the blueprints of life) to its offspring, which grows into a genetically identical duplicate of that parent.

Cloning Plants and Animals

The basic concept of cloning is nothing new. Indeed, both plants and animals have been cloned for a long time. Nature developed efficient cloning techniques long before humanity came into being, beginning with the very first one-celled organisms that appeared on Earth more than 3 billion years ago. A vast array of microbes, including protozoa, bacteria, blue-green algae, and some yeasts, replicated themselves and continue to do so today by means of cloning. Nature then passed on this biological ability to a number of plants even after sexual reproduction came into being. For example, strawberries are among many plants that owe their continued existence to cloning. Each strawberry plant sends out a stem called a stolon, which moves along the ground until it manages to take root. When this happens, a new plant, which is genetically nearly identical to the parent plant, springs to life on that spot. Other examples of plants that naturally reproduce through cloning include blackberries, artichokes, ivy, water hyacinths, and a number of garden flowers, among them tulips. In addition, over time human gardeners and farmers learned how to clone a wide array of plants, including all manner of vines, fruits, and vegetables. In fact, a large proportion of the produce sold today in grocery stores around the world is grown with artificial cloning techniques.

Given the long-standing human ability to clone plants, it was perhaps inevitable that people would eventually desire to clone animals, too. The basic process was first suggested in the 1930s by Nobel Prize–winning biologist Hans Spiemann. In theory, he said, one could take an egg from a female animal, remove the genetic material from the egg's nucleus, and then replace it with genetic material from a cell belonging to a second animal. After the egg grows into an embryo, one could implant it into the uterus of a female of that species. And a few months later a clone of the second animal would be born. Attempts to create cloned animals, including frogs, using this process repeatedly failed until 1996, when scientists at the Roslin Institute in Scotland managed to create the world's first cloned animal, a sheep they named Dolly.

> "Cloned cattle have been used to harvest life-giving medical drugs produced in their blood."

Dolly's creation opened the floodgates of animal cloning. Within a decade scientists working in a number of countries around the world had managed to clone cows, bulls, horses, pigs, rabbits, mice, rats, cats, dogs, and even monkeys. Some of these animals—especially the rats and mice—are used for research purposes. Cloned cattle have been used to harvest life-giving medical drugs produced in their blood. And cats and dogs recently began to be cloned to fulfill a demand by people who desire to acquire physical duplicates of their deceased pets. (The process can duplicate only physical characteristics; personality, memories, and so forth cannot be reproduced through cloning.) Scientists have even begun to save endangered species by cloning the last living members of those species. According to a recent statement by the Human Genome Project:

In 2001, the first clone of an endangered wild animal was born, a wild ox called a gaur. . . . In 2001, scientists in Italy reported the successful cloning of a healthy baby mouflon, an endangered wild sheep. . . . Other endangered species that are potential candidates for cloning include the African bongo antelope, the Sumatran tiger, and the giant panda.[49]

Human Cloning: Initial Breakthroughs and Reactions

The success achieved in cloning plants and animals inevitably led both scientists and nonscientists to consider the possibility of cloning human beings. They reasoned that if complex mammals such as horses, cows, cats, dogs, and especially monkeys can be cloned, it might be only a matter of time before science developed the technology and skills needed to clone people. One reason cited for wanting to clone people was the desire of some parents to produce physical duplicates of their deceased children. Another potential motive frequently cited for cloning humans is to provide another method, in addition to adoption and in vitro fertilization, for infertile couples to have children.

With these and other goals in mind, some researchers began working on the preliminary steps of human cloning in the late 1990s. In December 1998 a team of researchers in Seoul, South Korea, managed to clone a human embryo consisting of a few cells; not long afterward, several other labs around the world repeated the experiment with equal success. Having created viable human embryos, the next logical step was to implant them in the uteruses of women and allow them to grow into babies.

But this did not happen. The Korean scientists proceeded to destroy the embryos they had created. Moreover, most scientists around the world became very reluctant to continue their human cloning projects and began redirecting their time and resources to other areas of research.

The primary reason for this self-imposed roadblock in human cloning projects was a palpable fear of adverse public reactions to and legal sanctions on such research. Indeed, from the instant that Dolly the cloned lamb sprang into existence in Scotland in the mid-1990s, loud public protests and international debates erupted over the morality of cloning humans. In the words of Princeton University biologist Lee M. Silver, a widely respected expert on cloning:

> Many people were terrified by the prospect [of human cloning]. Ninety percent of Americans polled within the first week after the story [of Dolly's birth] broke felt that human cloning should be banned. And the opinions of many media pundits, ethicists, and policy makers, though not unanimous, seemed to follow those of the general public. The idea that humans might be cloned was called "morally despicable," repugnant," "totally inappropriate," as well as "ethically wrong, socially misguided, and biologically mistaken."[50]

Debates over the Morality of Human Cloning

One of the core reasons for this widespread negative reaction to the notion of human cloning is that many people feel it goes against their religious or spiritual values. A common perception among members of most of the world's major religions is that human cloning might somehow interfere with God's plan or wishes. Following Dolly's birth, Pope John Paul II made a statement condemning human cloning. The National Bioethics Advisory Commission, a group that advises the U.S. president on the ethical uses of science, gave a similar opinion, advising that "human beings should not probe the fundamental secrets or mysteries of life, which belong to God."[51]

Another common ethical argument against human cloning is that it could potentially be psychologically damaging, as well as socially and morally demeaning, for the person who is cloned. The World Health Organization takes this position, stating:

> Cloning . . . [has] unprecedented ethical implications and raise[s] serious concerns for the safety of

> " A common perception among members of most of the world's major religions is that human cloning might somehow interfere with God's plan or wishes. "

individuals and subsequent generations of human beings. . . . The use of cloning . . . for the replication of
human individuals is ethically unacceptable and contrary to human dignity and integrity.[52]

William Saunders, senior fellow in bioethics and human rights coun-
sel for the Family Research Council agrees, asking, "Would any of us
wish to live in a society where one class of human beings is manufactured
to suit the preferences of others?"[53]

> **[People] who are
> ethically unop-
> posed to cloning
> worry that im-
> portant scientific
> breakthroughs
> might never hap-
> pen if modern
> society does not
> develop the po-
> tential of human
> cloning.**

In response to such attacks on scientific exploration of human cloning,
some individuals and organizations argue that there is freedom both of and
from religion in the United States, as
well as freedom of speech and expres-
sion. And it would itself be unethical for one or more religious or other
groups to force society to adhere to
their personal moral views. Others
who are ethically unopposed to cloning worry that important scientific
breakthroughs might never happen if
modern society does not develop the
potential of human cloning. "We believe there is a very real danger that research with enormous potential benefits may be suppressed solely because it
conflicts with some people's religious beliefs," states the New York-based
International Academy of Humanism.

It is important to recognize that similar religious objections were once raised against autopsies, anesthesia, artificial insemination, and the entire genetic revolution of
our day—yet enormous benefits have accrued from each
of these developments.[54]

Brigitte Boisselier, scientific director of Clonaid, a controversial company offering to clone humans, makes a similar argument. "Centuries

ago, twins were killed because primitive people thought they were evil," she says, "Today ethicists are telling you the same about cloned children, . . . cloning is giving life to a few individuals and cannot harm any one."[55]

A National Ban Still Uncertain

Those who disagree with cloning advocates and think that human cloning will be a bad thing often talk about legally banning it. In 1997 the U.S. National Bioethics Advisory Commission recommended that laws be passed that would restrict and outlaw human cloning technology. A number of countries across the globe have already banned all human cloning research, among them the United Kingdom, Germany, Denmark, Australia, and Japan. A few states, including California and Michigan, have also imposed legal bans on human cloning. However, the U.S. federal government has not yet passed national legislation outlawing it, although it has forbidden federal funds from being used for such research.

> " A number of countries across the globe have already banned all human cloning research. "

The fact that no countrywide ban has yet been adopted in the United States has not stopped numerous leaders, Democrats and Republicans alike, from pushing for such a law. In 2002, for instance, President George W. Bush declared:

> Human cloning is deeply troubling to me, and to most Americans. Life is a creation, not a commodity. Our children are gifts to be loved and protected, not products to be designed and manufactured. . . . Fortunately, nearly every American agrees that [human cloning] should be banned.[56]

In spite of such widely accepted sentiments, at present the advent of a national ban on human cloning remains uncertain. And some people argue that such a ban goes against the democratic values making up the country's political, legal, and moral foundations. "Even if human cloning offers no obvious benefits to humanity, why ban it?" asks Ruth Macklin, a professor of bioethics at the Albert Einstein College of Medicine in New York City. "In a democratic society, we don't usually pass laws outlawing something before there is actual or probable evidence of harm."[57]

Macklin and a number of other thoughtful bioethicists argue instead for a sort of legal middle ground. This would consist of society's taking at least a few more years to think about the issue rationally and then proceeding with human cloning in a measured, tightly regulated manner. "A moratorium on further research into human cloning might make sense," Macklin writes:

> In order to consider calmly the grave questions it raises. If the moratorium is then lifted, human cloning should remain a research activity for an extended period. And if it is ever attempted, it should—and no doubt will—take place only with careful scrutiny and layers of legal oversight.[58]

Only time will tell whether American society will accept this compromise or, instead, will finally make human cloning illegal.

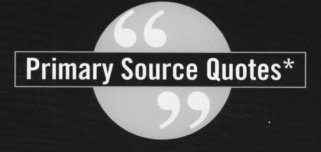

Primary Source Quotes*

Should Human Cloning Be Banned?

❝I believe human cloning is deeply troubling, and I strongly support efforts by Congress to ban all human cloning. We must advance the promise and cause of medical science. . . yet we must do so in ways that respect human dignity and help build a culture of life.**❞**

—George W. Bush, statement on House of Representatives action on legislation to prohibit human cloning, February 27, 2003. www.whitehouse.gov.

Bush is the forty-third president of the United States.

❝Every individual and his/her life experience is unique. . . . I should think any clone would treasure the gift of life and if raised in a normal environment, have the opportunity to cultivate his/her own personality just like any other person.**❞**

—Hsien Hsien Lei, "Your Genetic Clone's Individuality," *Genetics and Health*, July 17, 2006. www.geneticsandhealth.com.

Lei writes and edits numerous columns, including "Genetics and Health," for blogging network b5media.

* Editor's Note: While the definition of a primary source can be narrowly or broadly defined, for the purposes of Compact Research, a primary source consists of: 1) results of original research presented by an organization or researcher; 2) eyewitness accounts of events, personal experience, or work experience; 3) first-person editorials offering pundits' opinions; 4) government officials presenting political plans and/or policies; 5) representatives of organizations presenting testimony or policy.

Primary Source Quotes

❝Using technology [such as cloning] to alter nature is a requirement of human life. It is what brought man from the cave to civilization.❞

—Alex Epstein, "Cloning Is Moral," *Ayn Rand Institute*, February 13, 2004. www.aynrand.org.

Epstein is a writer for the Ayn Rand Institute, an organization dedicated to promoting the principles of individual rights.

❝Human cloning for reproduction is wrong. . . . Cloning would put scientists in the role of manufacturers, while people who were cloned would be reduced to the status of products or commodities.❞

—Brian Harradine, "Beware the Push for Human Cloning," *Age*, July 31, 2004. www.theage.com.

Harradine is an independent senator for Tasmania, Australia.

❝There are . . . times when the only course to prevent profound wrongs is to establish firm ethical and legal barriers beyond which we will not tread. Human cloning is such an issue."

—Wesley J. Smith, "Ian Wilmut: Human Cloner," *Weekly Standard*, February 16, 2005. www.weeklystandard.com.

Smith is a senior fellow at the Discovery Institute and a special consultant to the Center for Bioethics and Culture.

❝The real crime against Humanity is to deny the right to live forever [through human cloning].❞

—Brigitte Boisselier, "Human Discussion on Cloning at the UN," *Clonaid*, October 21, 2004. www.clonaid.com.

Boisselier is scientific director for Clonaid, a private company working to make human cloning a reality.

66 **Would being a clone be psychologically harmful? Would a clone feel destined to repeat the choices and behaviors of his progenitor? No . . . not any more than might occur with children of high-achieving or famous parents.** 99

—Arlene Judith Klotzko, "Is It Time to Allow Human Cloning? No—But Purely Because It Is Not Yet Safe," *Edge*, June 2004, pp. 18–19.

Klotzko is a bioethicist and lawyer and writes a weekly column called Science Matters for *Financial Times Magazine*.

66 **Member States [of the United Nations] are called upon to prohibit all forms of human cloning inasmuch as they are incompatible with human dignity and the protection of human life.** 99

—United Nations, "United Nations Declaration on Human Cloning," March 8, 2005. http://daccessdds.un.org.

The United Nations is an international organization established in 1945 to promote international law, security, and economic development.

66 **Cloning would allow us to hold on to those rarely occurring . . . [people] like Albert Einstein and give them additional lifetimes to use their unique talents and abilities. Cloning will enable humanity to retain its very best.** 99

—Randolfe H. Wicker, "Why Not Clone? Commentary on the Foregoing," *Clone Rights United Front*, February 3, 2003. www.clonerights.com.

Wicker is founder of Clone Rights United Front, an organization in favor of human cloning.

66 **Proponents of cloning want to usurp God's role and become creators and gods themselves, making off-spring in their own images. We were created to love and respect our Creator, not to attempt to be creators ourselves.** 99

—Joseph Candel, "Playing God? Facts and Thoughts on Human Cloning," *Activated*, July 2003. www.activatedminis tries.org.

Candel is a contributing writer to *Activated*, a monthly Christian magazine.

66 **Opposition to human cloning springs from . . . the fear . . . [that] 'We can't play God.' But why can't we? . . . A surgeon 'plays God' whenever he removes a cancer . . . rather than letting the patient die.** 99

—Harry Binswanger, "Immoral to Ban Human Cloning," *Ayn Rand Institute*, December 18, 2003. www.aynrand.org.

Binswanger teaches philosophy at the Ayn Rand Institute and is the author of *The Biological Basis of Teleological Concepts*.

66 **The case for banning human reproductive cloning is not difficult to make, at least for now. Most scientists agree that it is unsafe and likely to lead to serious ab-normalities and birth defects.** 99

—Michael J. Sandel, "The Ethical Implications of Human Cloning," *Perspectives in Biology and Medicine*, Spring 2005.

Sandel is a political philosopher.

Should Human Cloning Be Banned?

- In 1952 the first animal, a tadpole, was cloned.

- A number of specimens of endangered species have been cloned, including a gaur (wild ox) and a mouflon (wild sheep), taking science a step closer to human cloning.

- The first cloned human embryo was produced in the labs of Advanced Cell Technology, in Worcester, Massachusetts, in October 2001.

- More than 90 percent of cloning attempts fail to produce viable offspring.

- About 30 percent of clones born alive are affected with "large offspring syndrome" and other debilitating conditions.

- According to a major poll taken in 2001, 69 percent of Americans believe that human cloning is against God's will, while 23 percent think it is not.

- In 2002, researchers at the Whitehead Institute for Biomedical Research in Cambridge, Massachusetts, reported that the genomes of cloned mice were compromised. In analyzing more than 10 thousand liver and placenta cells of cloned mice, they discovered that about 4 percent of genes function abnormally.

Cloning a Human Being

Human cloning requires a female egg and a body cell such as a muscle or hair cell. The genes are removed from the egg cell and replaced with the body cell genes. The egg becomes an embryo and eventually develops into a clone of the person from which the body cell was taken. Unlike sexual reproduction, which combines the genes of two people, cloning reproduces the genes of one individual.

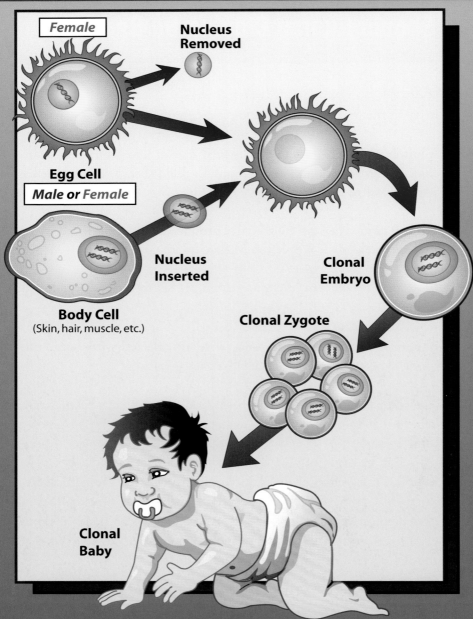

Female

Nucleus Removed

Egg Cell

Male or Female

Nucleus Inserted

Body Cell
(Skin, hair, muscle, etc.)

Clonal Embryo

Clonal Zygote

Clonal Baby

Source: Association of Reproductive Health Professionals, 2003.

- On March 17, 2005, the Human Cloning Prohibition Act of 2005, which was passed by the U.S. House of Representatives, was sent to the U.S. Senate.

- In May 2005, members of the United Nations General Assembly voted by a margin of 84 to 34 for a declaration calling on all nations to legally ban human cloning.

How Americans Feel About Animal Versus Human Cloning

While the majority of Americans are morally against cloning, more people approve of the cloning of animals than humans. Since 2001, those who feel it is morally acceptable to clone humans have risen from 7 percent to 9 percent, indicating a trend in public acceptance of cloning.

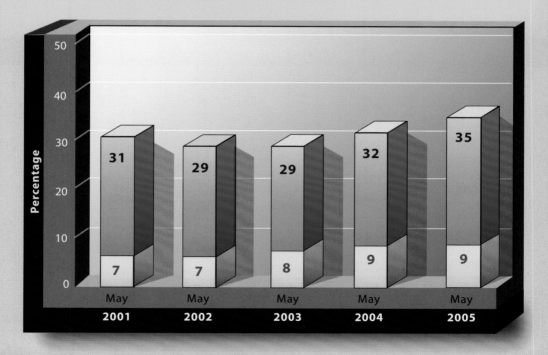

Morally acceptable to clone animals
Morally acceptable to clone humans

Source: The Gallup Organization, 2005.

Men More Likely than Women to Support Legalized Human Cloning

While 9 percent of the American public supports the legalization of human cloning, men are nearly three times as likely as women to support legalization. Opponents of human cloning stress that it is unethical, while supporters frequently cite that it allows infertile couples to have children.

Should human cloning be legal?

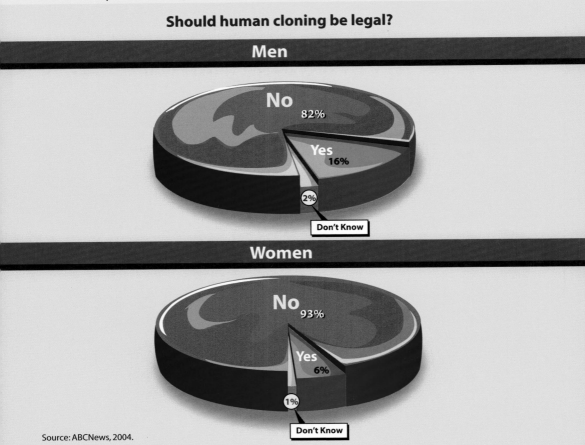

Men

No 82%

Yes 16%

2%

Don't Know

Women

No 93%

Yes 6%

1%

Don't Know

Source: ABCNews, 2004.

- Dolly, a sheep and the first mammal to be cloned from adult DNA, was euthanized by lethal injection February 14, 2003. Dolly had been suffering from lung cancer and crippling arthritis.

Key People and Advocacy Groups

Daniel Callahan: In 1969 Callahan cofounded the Hastings Center, a nonpartisan, nonprofit research institute dedicated to the exploration of questions in the fields of biomedical ethics, biotechnology, and the environment. He is currently the director of the center's International Program, as well as a senior fellow at Harvard Medical School.

Arthur Caplan: A world-renowned bioethicist, Caplan is Emanuel and Robert Hart professor of bioethics and director of the Center for Bioethics at the University of Pennsylvania. He is also the author or editor of 25 books, including *Finding Common Ground: Ethics and Assisted Suicide* (2001) and a regular commentator on MSNBC.com and television news programs.

Patrick Dixon: Dixon is the founder and chairman of Global Change Ltd. and a fellow of the Center for Management at London Business School. Often called one of Europe's leading futurists and commentators on bioethical issues, Dixon has authored twelve books, including *The Genetic Revolution.*

William B. Hurlbut: Hurlbut is a consulting professor of neurology and neurological sciences at Stanford Medical Center, Stanford University, and a current member of the President's Council on Bioethics. Hurlbut's areas of interest and expertise include the ethical issues associated with advancing biomedical technology, the biological basis of moral awareness, and studies in the integration of theology and the philosophy of biology.

Leon Kass: A distinguished bioethicist and a member and past chairman of the President's Council on Bioethics (2002–2005), Kass is presently the Addie Clark Harding Professor in the Committee on Social Thought and the College at the University of Chicago. Kass has also published numerous articles and several books, among them *The Challenge for Bioethics.*

Jack Kevorkian: Both widely hated and widely admired, Kevorkian was a staunch advocate of physician-assisted suicide who gained international recognition in the 1990s. According to his lawyer Geoffrey Fieger, the Michigan physician assisted in the suicide of almost one hundred terminally ill people between 1990 and 1998. In 1999 Kevorkian was tried and convicted of second-degree murder for helping Thomas Youk voluntarily end his life, and was sentenced to a ten- to twenty-five-year prison sentence. Kevorkian recently revealed that he is terminally ill with hepatitis C and is seeking a pardon, parole, or commutation of his sentence.

Robert M. Nelson: A frequent commentator on bioethical issues, Nelson is an attending intensivist (a doctor who specializes in the care of critically ill patients, usually those in an intensive care unit) and chairman of Children's Hospital of Philadelphia's institutional review board. Nelson is also the chairman of the Pediatric Advisory Committee of the U.S. Food and Drug Administration and holds a master of divinity degree from Yale Divinity School and a doctorate in the study of religion from Harvard University. A devout Christian, Nelson brings a strong religious perspective to current bioethical debates.

Edmund Pellegrino: Currently chairman of the President's Council on Bioethics, Pellegrino is a founding editor of the *Journal of Medicine and Philosophy* and is also the author or coauthor of twenty-four books and numerous articles dealing with medical and bioethical issues. Professor emeritus of medicine and medical ethics and adjunct professor of philosophy at Georgetown University, he has served as president and chairman of the Yale–New Haven Medical Center. In 2004 he was named to the International Bioethics Committee of the United Nations Education, Scientific, and Cultural Organization (UNESCO).

Harold T. Shapiro: Shapiro is a former president of Princeton University and a professor emeritus in the departments of economics and public policy at that institution. He was also the chairman of the National Bioethics Advisory Commission during President Bill Clinton's second term, when the organization's famous 2000 report on stem cell research was issued.

Lee M. Silver: A world-renowned expert on stem cells and cloning, Silver is a professor at Princeton University in the Department of Molecular Biology and the Woodrow Wilson School of Public and International Affairs. He has written numerous articles and books, including the best-selling *Remaking Eden* and the 2006 release *Challenging Nature: The Clash of Science and Spirituality at the New Frontiers of Life.*

Chronology

1996
Dolly the sheep, the first mammal cloned using adult cells, is born at the Roslin Institute in Scotland.

1953
Working at the Cavendish Labs in Cambridge, England, scientists Francis Crick and James Watson discover the structure of DNA, the primary chemical making up genes.

1990–2003
The U.S. Department of Energy and the U.S. National Institutes of Health conduct the Human Genome Project (HGP), in which scientists locate and identify almost thirty thousand genes in human DNA.

ca. 410–400 B.C.
The Greek physician Hippocrates and the members of his medical school reject the idea of physician-assisted suicide and formulate the Hippocratic Oath.

A.D.

400 B.C.   1910   1920   1930   1940   1950   1960   1970   1980   1990

1910
Thomas H. Morgan of Columbia University proves that genes are attached to chromosomes and that the positions of genes can be mapped, opening the way for later major developments in the science of genetics, including genetic screening.

1952
The first animal, a tadpole, is cloned.

1963
English biologist J.B.S. Haldane coins the term "clone."

1997
Oregon voters reject the challenges to the Death with Dignity Act, making Oregon the only state that allows physician-assisted suicide.

President Bill Clinton proposes legislation to ban human cloning for at least five years.

1994
Oregon's legislature passes the state's first Death with Dignity Act, allowing physician-assisted suicide, but the law immediately faces legal challenges.

Chronology

1998

Jack Kevorkian, a controversial figure in the "right-to-die" debate, appears on the television program *60 Minutes* and airs a video of one of his patients committing suicide.

Nineteen European countries sign a ban on human cloning.

Scientists at the University of Wisconsin and Johns Hopkins University become the first to isolate and grow human embryonic stem cells.

2006

In the first veto issued in his presidency, Bush quashes legislation passed by Congress that would have lifted the restrictions on federal funding of embryonic stem cell research.

2001

In a controversial move, President George W. Bush allows only a few existing stem cell lines to receive research funding.

The first cloned human embryo is produced in the labs of Advanced Cell Technology in Worcester, Massachusetts.

1998 1999 2000 2001 2002 2003 2004 2005 2006

1999

Kevorkian is convicted of murder for aiding others to commit suicide and begins serving a ten- to twenty-five-year sentence in a Michigan prison.

2004

Fifty-nine percent of Californians vote to pass Proposition 71, which earmarks $3 billion over ten years for stem cell research.

2005

A Death with Dignity act is introduced in Vermont's legislature but is not adopted into law.

Jack Kevorkian attempts but fails to gain parole.

A group of South Korean scientists produces the world's first cloned dog, fueling worries among various individuals and groups that cloning humans might occur in the near future.

2002

Australia's Parliament authorizes the use of new human stem cell lines for research.

Related Organizations

American Association for the Advancement of Science (AAAS)

Center for Science, Technology, and Congress

1200 New York Ave. NW

Washington, DC 20005

phone: (202) 326-6400

Web site: www.aaas.org

Established as the Center for Science, Technology, and Congress in July 1994 and funded by a grant from the Burroughs Welcome Fund, the center provides information to Congress on current science and technology issues and assistance to the science and engineering community in understanding and working with Congress. The center publishes the newsletter *Science and Technology in Congress* monthly when Congress is in session.

American Society of Law, Medicine and Ethics

765 Commonwealth Ave., Suite 1634

Boston, MA 02215

phone: (617) 262-4990

fax: (617) 437-7596

Web site: www.aslme.org

The mission of the American Society of Law, Medicine and Ethics is to provide scholarship, debate, and critical thought to professionals in the areas of law, medicine, and ethics. The organization also provides information to the public on a wide range of bioethical issues, including physician-assisted suicide.

Center for Science in the Public Interest

1875 Connecticut Ave. NW, Suite 300

Washington, DC 20009

phone: (202) 332-9110

fax: (202) 265-4954

Web site: www.cspinet.org

The Center for Science in the Public Interest is a consumer advocacy organization whose missions are to conduct research and advocacy programs in health and nutrition and to provide consumers with current information about health and well-being.

Christian Medical and Dental Associations

PO Box 7500

2604 Hwy. 421

Bristol, TN 37621

phone: (423) 844-1000 or (888) 230-2637

fax: (423) 844-1005

Web site: www.cmawashington.org

The Christian Medical and Dental Associations' stated mission is to motivate, educate, and equip Christian physicians and dentists to glorify God. It seeks to advance biblical principles in bioethics and health to the church and society at large. Among its publications is the quarterly magazine *Today's Christian Doctor* and the monthly newsletter *Scan.*

Compassion & Choices

PO Box 101810

Denver, CO 80250-1810

phone: (800) 247-7421

fax: (303) 639-1224

Web site: www.compassionandchoices.org

Compassion & Choices is the largest end-of-life advocacy organization in the United States. It provides education and advocacy for patients and their families, as well as medical personnel, facing end-of-life decisions. It publishes the quarterly magazine *Compassion and Choices.*

Dying with Dignity

55 Eglinton Ave. East, Suite 802

Toronto, Ontario M4P 1G8

Canada

phone: (416) 486-3998 or 800-495-6156

fax: (416) 486-5562

e-mail: info@dyingwithdignity.ca

Web site: www.dyingwithdignity.ca

The stated objective of this charitable organization is to improve the quality of dying for all Canadians. It provides education about health care options at the end of life including living wills and enduring powers of attorney for personal care. It publishes a quarterly newsletter, *Dying with Dignity.*

The Hastings Center

21 Malcolm Gordon Rd.

Garrison, NY 10524-4125

phone: (845) 424-4040

fax: (845) 424-4545

Web site: www.thehastingscenter.org

The Hastings Center is an independent, nonpartisan, and nonprofit bioethics research institute founded in 1969 to explore issues in health care, biotechnology, and the environment. It provides information about nearly all bioethical issues, including stem cells, genetic testing, and cloning, and publishes the bimonthly journal *Hastings Center Report.*

National Human Genome Research Institute

Communications and Public Liaison Branch

National Institutes of Health

Bldg. 31, Room 4B09

31 Center Dr. MSC 2152

9000 Rockville Pike

Bethesda, MD 20892-2152

phone: (301) 402-0911

fax: (301) 402-2218

Web site: www.genome.gov

The institute is the primary National Institutes of Health (NIH) organization for information about research on genetic testing, cloning, stem cell research, and other scientific issues with ethical ramifications.

National Library of Medicine (NLM)

8600 Rockville Pike

Bethesda, MD 20894

phone: (301) 594-5983 or (888) 346-3656

fax: (301) 408-1384

Web site: www.nlm.nih.gov

The National Library of Medicine (NLM), on the campus of the National Institutes of Health in Bethesda, Maryland, is the world's largest medical library. It collects materials and provides information and research services in all areas of biomedicine and health care; assists the advancement of medical and related sciences through the collection, dissemination, and exchange of information important to the progress of medicine and health; and serves as a national information resource for medical education, research, and service activities of federal and private agencies, organizations, and institutions.

National Newborn Screening and Genetics Resource Center (NNSGRC)

1912 W. Anderson Ln., Suite 210

Austin, TX 78757

phone: (512) 454-6419

fax: (512) 454-6509

Web site: http://genes-r-us.uthscsa.edu

The NNSGRC provides information and resources in the area of newborn screening and genetics to health professionals, the public health community, consumers, and government officials.

President's Council on Bioethics

1801 Pennsylvania Ave. NW, Suite 700

Washington, DC 20006

phone: (202) 296-4669

Web site: www.bioethics.gov

The President's Council on Bioethics is charged with advising the president of the United States on bioethical issues that may emerge as a consequence of advances in biomedical science and technology, such as embryo and stem cell research, assisted reproduction, cloning, enhancement of human capacities through genetics and the neurosciences, and end-of-life issues. Recent publications include *Taking Care: Ethical Caregiving in Our Aging Society, Reproduction and Responsibility: The Regulation of New Biotechnologies,* and *Monitoring Stem Cell Research.*

For Further Research

Books

Michael Cuse and Christopher A. Pynes, *The Stem Cell Controversy: Debating the Issues.* New York: Prometheus, 2006.

David Goodnough, *The Debate over Human Cloning.* Berkley Heights, NJ: Enslow, 2003.

Suzanne Holland et al., eds., *The Human Embryonic Stem Cell Debate: Science, Ethics, and Public Policy.* Cambridge, MA: MIT Press, 2002.

Carol Levine, *Taking Sides: Clashing Views on Controversial Bioethical Issues.* New York: McGraw-Hill, 2005.

Jane Maenschein, *Whose View of Life? Embryos, Cloning, and Stem Cells.* Cambridge, MA: Harvard University Press, 2003.

Joseph Panno, *Stem Cell Research: Medical Applications and Ethical Controversy.* New York: Facts On File, 2004.

Barry Rosenfeld, *Assisted Suicide and the Right to Die.* Washington, DC: American Psychological Association, 2004.

Margaret A. Sommerville, *Death Talk: The Case Against Euthanasia and Physician-Assisted Suicide.* Quebec: McGill Queen's University Press, 2002.

Henk Ten Have et al., *The Ethics of Genetic Screening.* New York: Springer, 2002.

Robert M. Veatch, *The Basics of Bioethics.* Upper Saddle River, NJ: Prentice Hall, 2000.

Brent Waters and Ronald Cole-Turner, eds., *God and the Embryo: Religious Voices on Stem Cells and Cloning.* Washington, DC: Georgetown University Press, 2003.

Periodicals

Mary Carmichael, "Eggs, Lies, Stem Cells," *Newsweek,* December 5, 2005.

Gareth Cook, "Paper Details Failed Human Cloning Attempts," *Boston Globe,* July 21, 2006.

Gregg Easterbrook, "Medical Evolution: Will Homo Sapiens Become Obsolete?" *New Republic,* February 17, 2000.

Nancy Gibbs, "Stem Cells: The Hope and the Hype," *Time,* August 7, 2006.

Lawrence O. Gostin, "Physician-Assisted Suicide: A Legitimate Modern Practice?" *Journal of the American Medical Association,* April 26, 2006.

Bernadine Healy, "To Create or Not to Create," *U.S. News & World Report,* March 21, 2005.

Claudia Kalb and Debra Rosenberg, "Stem Cell Division," *Newsweek,* October 25, 2004.

Noelle Knox, "An Agonizing Debate About Euthanasia," *USA Today,* November 22, 2005.

Steve Lebau and Richard Neuworth, "Genetic Testing: Balancing Benefits and Abuses," *USA Today,* July 8, 2000.

Gilbert Meilaender, "Designing Our Descendants," *First Things,* January 2001.

New York Times, "The Rights of the Terminally Ill," May 28, 2004.

Paul Raeburn et al., "Everything You Need to Know About Cloning," *Business Week,* April 29, 2002.

Seth Stern and Jacqui Goddard, "The Murky Side of Right-to-Die Laws," *Christian Science Monitor,* October 13, 2003.

John Swartz and James Estin, "In Oregon, Choosing Death over Suffering," *New York Times,* June 1, 2004.

Margaret Talbot, "A Desire to Duplicate," *New York Times Magazine,* February 4, 2001.

Andrew E. Wurmaser and Fred H. Gage, "Stem Cells: Cell Fusion Causes Confusion," *Nature,* April 4, 2002.

Internet Sources

Arthur Caplan, "Cloning Ethics: Separating the Science from Fiction." http://msnbc.msn.com/id/3076920.

Global Change.com, "Future of Stem Cell Research: Rapid Progress." www.globalchange.com/stemcells2.htm.

Diane N. Irving, "Playing God by Manipulating Man: The Facts and Frauds of Human Cloning." www.mocatholic.org/Agenda/Irving Cloning.pdf.

Jeffrey P. Kahn, "Genetic Testing and Insurance." www.cnn.com/HEALTH/bioethics/9808/genetics.part2/template.html.

New Scientist.com, "First Cloned Pet Revives Ethical Debate." www.newscientist.com/article.ns?id=dn6833.

Source Notes

Overview: Questions of Morality in a Technological Age

1. Anna Tilley, "Bioethics," *Biomedical Scientist*, June 2001. www.ibms.org.
2. Chris Rangel, "When Doctors and Hospitals Decide to Pull the Plug," *RangelMD.com*, February 18, 2005. www.rangelmd.com.
3. Nancy S. Jecker and Lawrence J. Schneiderman, "Stopping Futile Medical Treatment: Ethical Issues," in David C. Thomasma, ed., *Birth to Death: Science and Bioethics*. New York: Cambridge University Press, 1996, p. 44.
4. Arthur Caplan, "The Time Has Come to Let Terri Schiavo Die," *Bioethics. net*, March 18, 2005. www.bioethics. net.
5. Laurie Zoloth, "The Necessary Conversation," *Beliefnet*. www.beliefnet.com.
6. Catherine Baker, *Your Genes, Your Choices*, Oak Ridge National Laboratory. www.ornl.gov.
7. Bill Muehlenberg, "Cloning Concerns," *Australian Family*, April 2000. www.family.org.au.
8. Clone Rights United Front, "Mission Statement." www.clonerights.com.
9. Kevin Bonsor, "How Designer Children Will Work," *HowStuffWorks*. www. howstuffworks.com.
10. Nicholas Agar, "Designer Babies: Ethical Considerations," ActionBioscience.org, April 2006. www.action bioscience.org.

Is Physician-Assisted Suicide Ethical?

11. American Geriatrics Society, "Physician-Assisted Suicide and Voluntary Active Euthanasia," November 2002. www. americangeriatrics.org.
12. Quoted in Barry Rosenfeld, *Assisted Suicide and the Right to Die*. Washington, DC: American Psychological Association, 2004, p. 16.
13. Noelle Knox, "An Agonizing Debate About Euthanasia," *USA Today*, November 22, 2005. www.usatoday.com.
14. Robert B. Mellert, "Cure or Care: The Future of Medical Ethics," *Futurist*, July/August 1997.
15. Kathryn L. Tucker, testimony before the Senate Judiciary Committee, Subcommittee on the Constitution, Civil Rights, and Property Rights, "The Consequences of Legalized Assisted Suicide and Euthanasia," May 25, 2006.www.compassionandchoices.org.
16. Quoted in James Kirkpatrick, "Supreme Court Will Rule on Euthanasia," *Conservative Chronicle*, October 30, 1996.
17. Peter Singer, "Decisions About Death," *Free Inquiry*, August/September 2005.
18. Richard Radtke, "A Case Against Physician-Assisted Suicide," *Journal of Disability Policy Studies*, Summer 2005.
19. Stolinsky, "Assisted Suicide of the Medical Profession," Stolinsky.com, March 20, 2006. www.stolinsky.com.
20. Eric Cohen and Leon R. Kass, " 'Cast Me Not Off in Old Age,' " *Commentary*, January 2006.
21. Stolinsky, "Assisted Suicide of the Medical Profession."
22. Wesley J. Smith, testimony before the Senate Judiciary Committee Subcommittee on the Constitution, Civil Rights, and Property Rights, "The Consequences of Legalized Assisted Suicide and Euthanasia, May 25, 2006. www.discovery.org.

Source Notes

23. John B. Feister, "Thou Shalt Not Kill: The Church Against Assisted Suicide," *St. Anthony Messenger,* June 1997. www.americancatholic.org.

24. B.A. Robinson, "Euthanasia and Physician Assisted Suicide," *Religious Tolerance,* November 7, 2001. www.religioustolerance.org/euth2.htm.

Are Some Kinds of Genetic Testing Unethical?

25. Lee M. Silver, *Remaking Eden: Cloning and Beyond in a Brave New World.* New York: Avon, 1997, p. 254.

26. George Neumayr, "The New Eugenics," *American Spectator*, July 13, 2005.

27. Neumayr, "The New Eugenics."

28. Catherine Baker, "Your Genes, Your Choices," Oak Ridge National Laboratory. www.ornl.gov.

29. Human Genetics Commission, "Choosing the Future: Genetics and Reproductive Decision-Making," July 2004. www.hgc.gov.uk.

30. Stephen Pinker, "The Designer Baby Myth," *Guardian*, June 5, 2003. www.guardian.co.uk.

31. Quoted in United States Conference of Catholic Bishops, "Critical Decisions: Genetic Testing and Its Implications," 1996. www.nccbuscc.org.

32. Karina Monteiro, "The Decision of Prenatal Genetic Testing," High School Bioethics Project, 2002. www.bioethics.upenn.edu.

33. Patrick Dixon, "Genetic Testing and Genetic Screening: Ethics of Genetic Testing for Insurance," Globalchange.com. www.globalchange.com.

34. Council for Responsible Genetics, "Genetic Discrimination," January 2001. www.gene-watch.org.

35. Arthur Caplan, "Ethics of Genetic Testing," keynote address, Second National Undergraduate Bioethics Conference, March 31, 2000. www.virginia.edu.

Should Human Embryos Be Used in Stem Cell Research?

36. Thomas B. Okarma, "Human Embryonic Stem Cells: A Primer on the Technology and Its Medical Applications," in Suzanne Holland et al., eds., *The Human Embryonic Stem Cell Debate: Science, Ethics, and Public Policy.* Cambridge, MA: MIT Press, 2002, p. 3.

37. Nancy Gibbs, "Stem Cells: The Hope and the Hype," *Time,* August 7, 2006, p. 42.

38. Quoted in Gregg Easterbrook, "Medical Evolution: Will Homo Sapiens Become Obsolete?" *New Republic,* February 17, 2000. www.freerepublic.com.

39. George W. Bush, "Message to the House of Representatives," July 19, 2006. www.whitehouse.gov.

40. Quoted in Gibbs, "Stem Cells," p. 43.

41. Easterbrook, "Medical Evolution."

42. Lawrence H. Summers, quoted in *Harvard University Gazette,* "Approval Granted for Harvard Stem Cell Researchers to Attempt Creation of Disease-Specific Embryonic Cell Lines," June 6, 2006. www.news.harvard.edu.

43. Hannah M. Vick, "Embryonic Stem Cell Research: Ethically Wrong Treatment of the Tiniest Humans," Concerned Women for America, May 1, 2000. www.cwfa.org.

44. Brian Harradine, "Beware the Push for Human Cloning," *Age*, July 31, 2004. www.theage.com.

45. Stem Cell Research Foundation, "Stem Cell Research: A Revolution in Medicine." www.stemcellresearchfoundation.org.

46. Quoted in Gibbs, "Stem Cells," p. 42.
47. Arthur Caplan, testimony before a subcommittee of the Senate Committee on Appropriations, "Stem Cell Research," 105th Cong., 2nd session. December 2, 1998. http://frwebgate. access.gpo.gov.
48. Margaret R. McLean, "Stem Cells: Shaping the Future in Public Policy," in Holland et al., *Human Embryonic Stem Cell Debate,* p. 205.

Should Human Cloning Be Banned?

49. Human Genome Project, "Cloning Fact Sheet," August 29, 2006. www. ornl.gov.
50. Lee M. Silver, *Remaking Eden: How Genetic Engineering and Cloning Will Transform the American Family.* New York: Avon, 1998, p. 108.
51. National Bioethics Advisory Commission, *Cloning Human Beings: Report and Recommendations,* Rockville, Maryland, 1997, pp. 45–46.
52. World Health Organization, "A Dozen Questions (and Answers) on Human Cloning." www.who.int.
53. William Saunders, testimony before the Health and Government Operations Committee of the Maryland House of Delegates, March 17, 2006. www.stemcellresearch.org.
54. International Academy of Humanism, "Declaration in Defense of Cloning," *Free Inquiry,* Summer 1997, pp. 11–12.
55. Brigitte Boisselier, "Human Discussion on Cloning at the UN," *Clonaid,* October 21, 2004. www.clonaid.com.
56. George W. Bush, "President Bush Calls on Senate to Back Human Cloning Ban," April 10, 2002. www.white house.gov.
57. Ruth Macklin, "Human Cloning? Don't Just Say No," *U.S. News & World Report,* March 10, 1997, p. 16.
58. Macklin, "Human Cloning?" p. 16.

List of Illustrations

Index

About the Author

In addition to his numerous acclaimed volumes on ancient civilizations, historian Don Nardo has published several studies of modern scientific discoveries, phenomena, and issues and their impact on society. Among these are *Ice Ages, Ozone, Vaccines, The Extinction of the Dinosaurs, Cloning, Black Holes,* and a biography of Charles Darwin. Mr. Nardo lives with his wife, Christine, in Massachusetts.